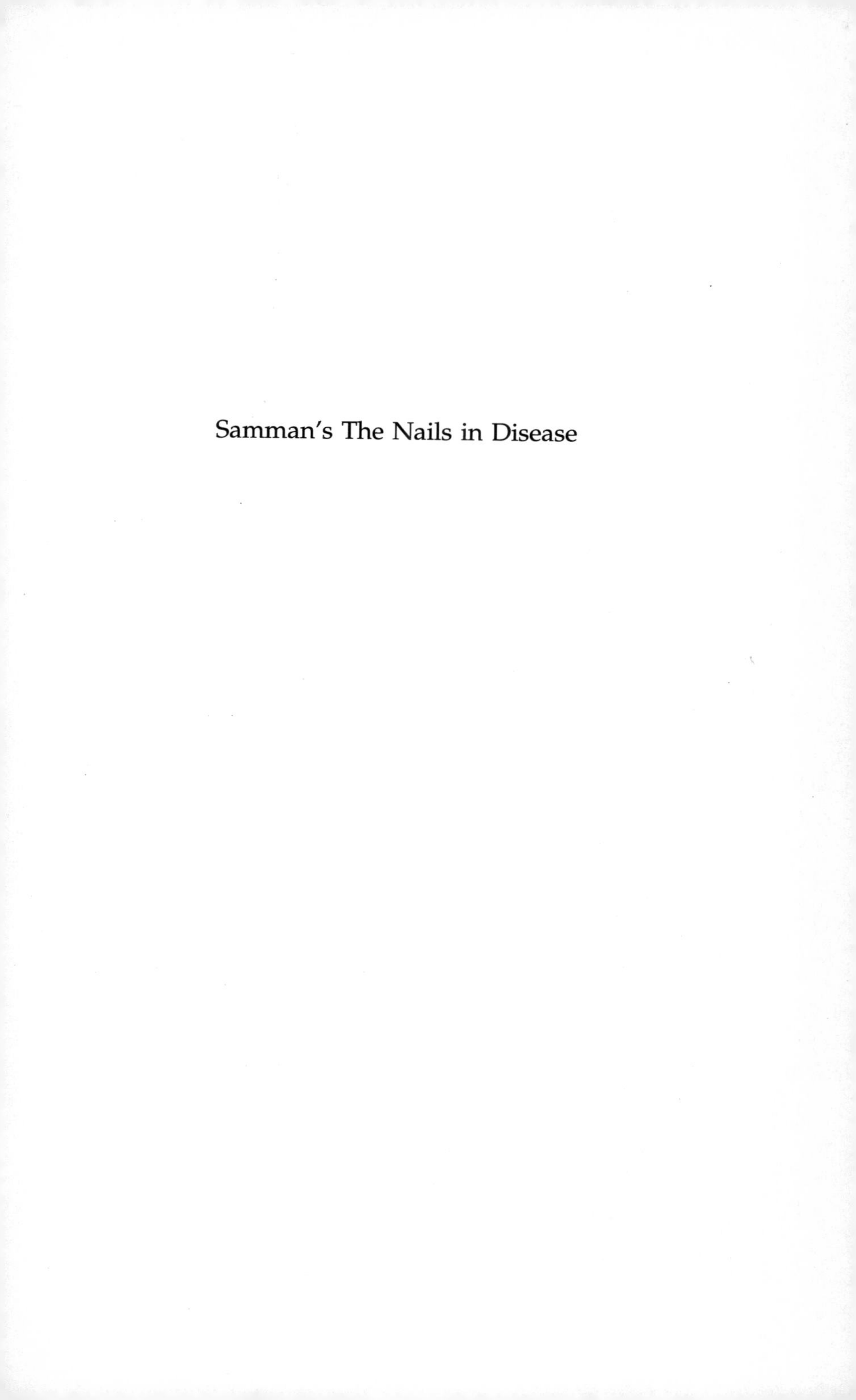

Samman's The Nails in Disease

Samman's
The Nails in Disease

Peter D. Samman
MA, MD, (Camb), FRCP (Lond)
Formerly Honorary Consultant Physician for Diseases of the Skin, Westminster Hospital and Honorary Consultant Physician to St John's Hospital for Diseases of the Skin

and

David A. Fenton
MB, ChB, (Liverpool), MRCP (UK)
St Thomas's Hospital, St John's Institute of Dermatology

Fifth Edition

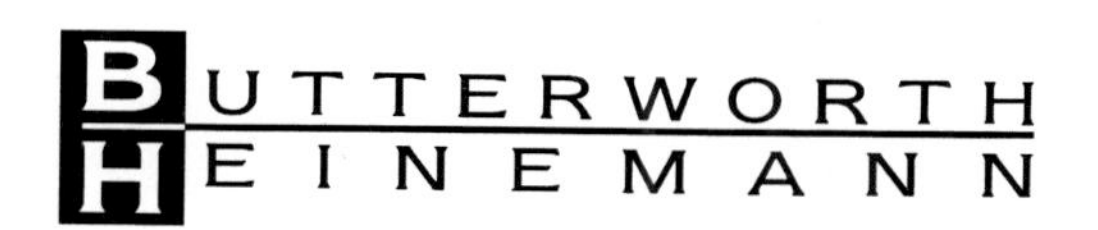

Butterworth-Heinemann Ltd
Linacre House, Jordan Hill, Oxford OX2 8DP

A member of the Reed Elsevier plc group

OXFORD LONDON BOSTON
MUNICH NEW DELHI SINGAPORE SYDNEY
TOKYO TORONTO WELLINGTON

First published 1965
Second edition 1972
Third edition 1978
Fourth edition 1986
Fifth edition 1995

British Library Cataloguing in Publication Data
Samman, Peter D.
Samman's Nails in Disease. – 5 Rev. ed
I. Title II. Fenton, David A.
616.547

ISBN 0 7506 0189 2

Library of Congress Cataloguing in Publication Data
Samman, Peter D. (Peter Derrick)
Samman's the nails in disease/Peter D. Samman and David A. Fenton. – 5th ed.
p. cm.
Rev. ed. of: The nails in disease. 4th ed. 1986.
Includes bibliographical references and index.
ISBN 0 7506 0189 2
1. Nail manifestations of general diseases. I. Fenton, David A. II. Samman, Peter D. (Peter Derrick). Nails in disease. III. Title. IV. Title: Nails in disease.
[DNLM: 1. Nail Diseases. 2. Nails. WR 475 S189s 1994]
RL 169.S25 1994
616.5'47—dc20
94-34926
CIP

Typeset by TecSet Ltd, Wallington, Surrey
Printed and bound in France

Contents

Contributors

R. Baran MD
Head of the Dermatological Unit, General Hospital, Cannes, France

R. P. R. Dawber MA, MB, ChB, FRCP
Consultant Dermatologist, Oxford Hospitals and Clinical Lecturer in Dermatology, University of Oxford

D. A. Fenton MB, ChB, MRCP
St John's Institute of Dermatology, St Thomas's Hospital

R. J. Hay DM, MRCP
Professor of Cutaneous Medicine, St John's Institute of Dermatology, Guy's Hospital

P. D. Samman MA, MD, FRCP
Formerly Honorary Consultant Physician for Diseases of the Skin, Westminster Hospital, and Honorary Consultant Physician to St John's Hospital for Diseases of the Skin

Preface to fifth edition

The Nails in Disease was conceived by Peter D. Samman in 1965, following a life-long interest in the study of nails and their disorders. I joined as co-author and co-editor for the fourth edition in 1986.

This updated and expanded fifth edition maintains and achieves the aims of the first, as a practical office guide to nail diseases and their management. It is intended for practising physicians, chiropodists and manicurists rather than research workers, and is written in a form which is easily understandable.

Most of the illustrations have now been replaced in full colour and I am grateful to those who have assisted with the task of providing new colour photographs, in particular to the Medical Illustration Departments of St John's Institute of Dermatology and St Thomas's Hospital.

I also extend my appreciation to numerous colleagues who continue to refer cases of nail disorders to me. Thanks to the staff of Butterworth-Heinemann for their continued encouragement and maintenance of quality and high standards.

Peter Derrick Samman died on 1st December 1992, during the preparation of this edition of his work. He was a quiet, highly respected gentleman of dermatology, who was always approachable, interested and stimulating.

The fifth edition of his book is dedicated to his memory.

D.A.F.

1

Anatomy and physiology

P. D. Samman

The chief function of the nail in man is that of protection. It protects the delicate terminal phalanx and greatly helps in the appreciation of fine touch and aids in picking up small objects. It is, of course, also used for scratching. A finger deprived of its nail is considerably less valuable than one possessing a nail and even the loss of a toe nail is the cause of some hardship. The main reason for complaint in nail deformities is, however, cosmetic. The nail is greatly modified in some mammals, for example, as a point of locomotion—the hoof, or as a prehensile organ—the claw.

Anatomy

The nail plate consists of hard keratin and is derived from an invagination of epidermis situated on the dorsum of the terminal phalanx. This invagination is first visible in the 9 week embryo and the formation of the nail is virtually complete by the 20th week (Zaias, 1963). A longitudinal section through the distal phalanx of a full term fetal toe is shown in Fig. 1.1.

The nail fold consists of a roof, a floor and lateral walls, while the nail bed represents that part of the dorsum of the terminal phalanx which lies below the exposed nail plate. There is some argument as to the area of the nail fold and nail bed which takes part in the formation of the nail plate.

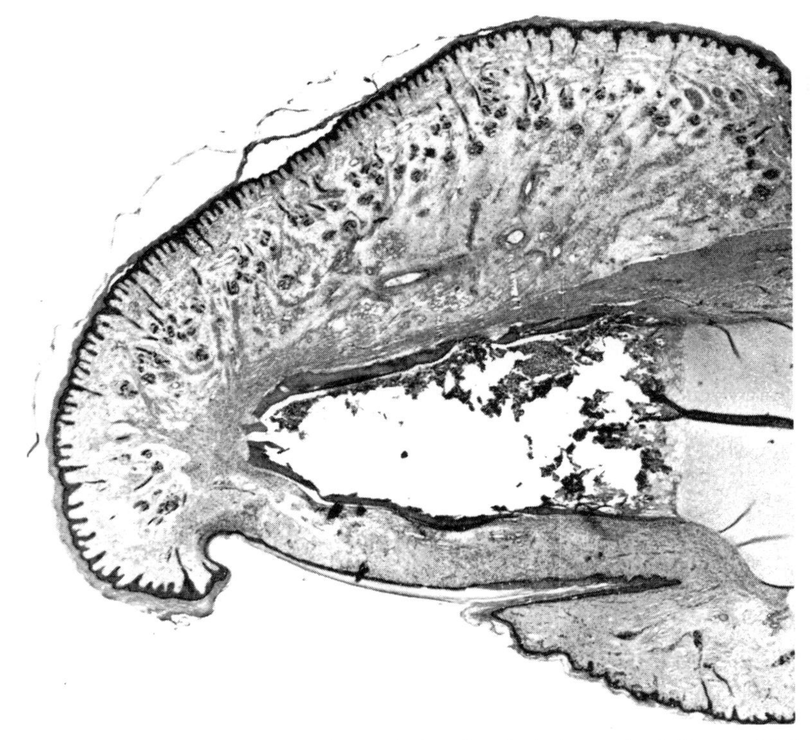

Fig. 1.1 Longitudinal section through the distal phalanx of a full term fetal toe (photomicrograph)

It is generally accepted that the nail plate is formed from the matrix. The matrix consists of the floor of the nail fold extending from the junction of floor and roof posteriorly to the anterior end of the lunula in front. The latter may or may not be visible but can usually be seen on the thumbs. It is paler than the remainder of the nail plate. It is probable that a small part of the roof of the nail fold also takes part of the formation of the nail plate.

The upper surface of the nail is formed from the most proximal portion of the matrix (including the roof of the nail fold when this contributes to the plate) while the lower surface is formed from the area close to the distal edge of the lunula. The nail bed itself is generally considered to take no part in the formation of the nail plate (Fig. 1.2(*a*)). This view was supported by Zaias and Alvarez (1968) in

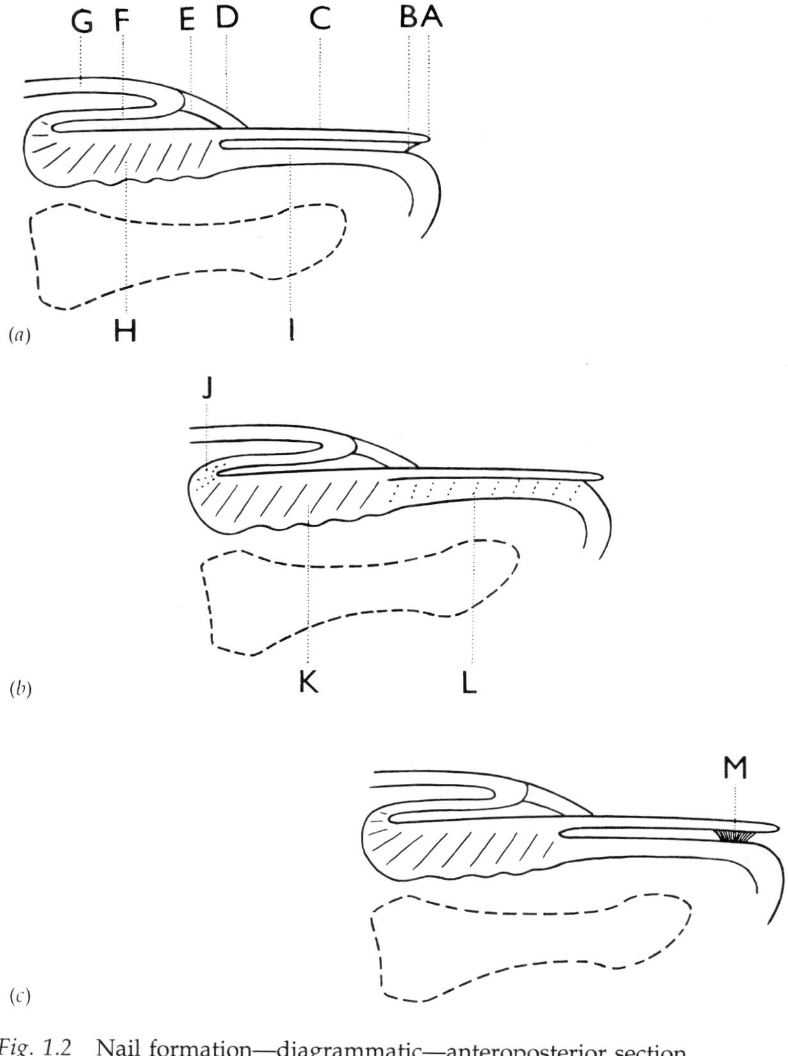

Fig. 1.2 Nail formation—diagrammatic—anteroposterior section

(*a*) Traditional theory
(*b*) Theory of Lewis
(*c*) Theory of Boas
A. Free margin of nail
B. Hyponychium
C. Nail plate
D. Cuticle
E. Eponychium
F. Roof of nail fold
G. Skin overlying posterior nail fold
H. Matrix
I. Nail bed
J. Matrix of dorsal nail
K. Matrix of intermediate nail
L. Matrix of ventral nail
M. Solenhorn

experiments on the squirrel monkey, a primate with a flat nail very similar to that of man. They showed by autoradiographic studies following the injection of tritiated glycine either intraperitoneally or into the tissues around the nail that the matrix alone supplied material to the nail plate. Later, similar experiments (Norton, 1971) on human volunteers, however, showed that there was some activity in the nail bed and so the formation of the nail in the squirrel monkey is somewhat different from that in humans.

Barton Lewis (1954) put forward the view that the nail is formed in three layers which he calls dorsal, intermediate and ventral nails. The intermediate nail is the main portion and is derived from the greater part of the (conventional) matrix; the dorsal nail is derived from the roof and a small portion of floor of the nail fold, while the ventral nail arises from the nail bed distal to the lunula (Fig. 1.2(*b*)). The lateral walls of the nail fold also contribute material to the nail plate. Although there is some doubt as to the validity of Lewis's theory there is no doubt that under pathological conditions material may at times be added to the nail plate from a large part of the nail bed and this fact is of importance in the interpretation of some nail disorders. Histochemical studies show that the material of the upper surface and that of the lower surface of the nail plate stains differently from the true hard keratin of the greater part of the nail (Achten, 1963; Jarrett and Spearman, 1966). The firm adhesion of the nail plate to the nail bed, although in part accounted for by corrugations on the under-surface of the nail plate fitting into similar corrugations on the nail bed, strongly suggests that the nail bed does contribute to the nail plate. The question of whether this material should be accepted as nail keratin is problematical. Achten (1972), for example, does not consider it to be true nail. These two opposing views of nail formation are illustrated diagrammatically in Figs. 1.2(*a*) and (*b*).

In mammals possessing a claw the matrix consists of two portions, one giving rise to the superficial stratum and the other to the deep stratum of the claw (Fig. 1.3). In the flat nail of most primates the deep stratum is lost and only the superficial stratum remains (le Gros Clark, 1959). The deep stratum, if it persisted, would correspond approximately to Lewis's ventral nail.

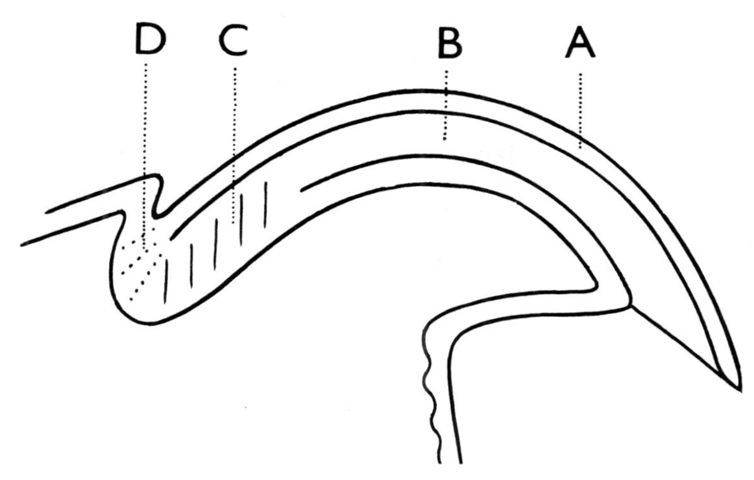

Fig. 1.3 Diagram of section through a mammalian claw—anteroposterior (Based on Clark)

A. Superficial stratum C. Terminal matrix
B. Deep stratum D. Basal matrix

Pinkus (1927) quotes Boas (1894) in describing the nail bed as consisting of three parts:

(1) The proximal part extending as far forward as the distal margin of the lunula, which is the nail-forming or fertile part of the nail bed.

(2) The part on which the nail lies and takes no part in the formation of the nail and is the sterile part of the nail bed; it extends from the distal margin of the lunula to the line where the anterior edge of the nail separates from the bed, the yellow line also known as the onychodermal band (Terry, 1955).

(3) The 'sole horn' (*sohlenhorn*) which again brings horny substance to the nail but does not form actual nail. This is the anterior fertile part or terminal matrix (Fig. 1.2(*c*)). It is perhaps this 'sole horn' which can become more extensive under pathological conditions, and may be the only vestige of the deep stratum (of the claw) normally present in humans. It is certainly not always present, even as a vestige, but is probably more often present on the toes than on the fingers. Its presence probably accounts for the appearance of spicules of nail which may form towards the tip of the digit after attempts at permanent ablation of the nail and matrix.

The author believes that all three modes of nail formation can occur on normal subjects, but that participation of much of the nail bed below the exposed nail is commoner in pathological than in healthy conditions.

Although the nail bed may at times take no part in the formation of the nail plate it is firmly attached to the nail bed, and if the nail is torn off the epidermis of the nail bed remains attached to the nail. It is probable that the epidermis of the nail bed moves forward with the growth of the nail. This epidermis is sometimes called the hyponychium; the latter term is at times used in a more restrictive sense to describe a forward extension of the epidermis of the floor of the nail fold on to the under-surface of the nail. Used in this way the term is more comparable with the use of the term eponychium (see below).

The cuticle is an extension of the epidermis (usually only the horny layer) of the smooth skin of the dorsum of the finger on to the nail plate, and it may extend quite a long way on to the nail (Figs. 1.2 and 1.4). If the cuticle is pushed back too roughly and cut, which often occurs if manicure is done clumsily, it is destroyed and this opens up the space between the nail plate and the roof of the nail fold.

The eponychium is an anterior extension of the roof of the nail fold on to the nail plate and also consists only of epidermis (Figs 1.2 and 1.4). It is of little importance clinically.

In the adult finger about a third of the nail plate is covered by the posterior fold and the matrix extends for 1–2 mm beyond the apparent commencement of the nail plate because the latter is extremely thin at its point of origin. The space between the matrix and the upper surface of the distal phalanx is very small.

The histology of the nail bed is similar to that of skin except that the epidermal layer is devoid of stratum lucidum and stratum granulosum and there are no secretory or pilosebaceous adnexae. The dermis of the nail bed is arranged in longitudinal grooves and ridges. The rete ridges (of the epidermis) are thin and project into the grooves of the dermis. The epidermis of the nail matrix is thick and passes gradually into the substance of the nail plate. The plate is formed by a series of changes similar to keratinisation of the epidermis, namely swelling of the cells followed by nucleolysis and subsequent shrinkage (Lewin, De Wit and Ferrington, 1972).

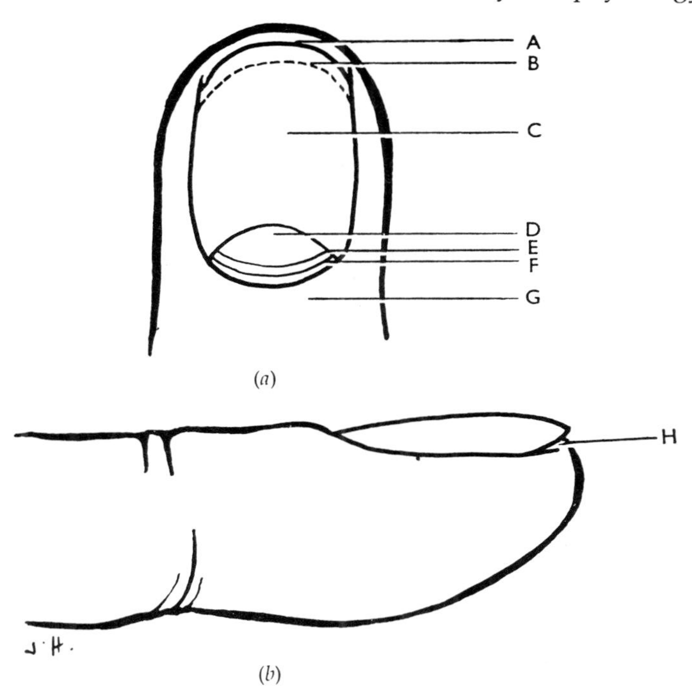

Fig. 1.4 Principal features of the nail (*a*) from above and (*b*) from the side (Diagram based on Pinkus, 1927)

A. Free margin of nail
B. Point of separation of nail from bed—'yellow line' or onychodermal band
C. Nail plate
D. Lunula
E. Cuticle
F. Eponychium
G. Skin overlying posterior nail fold
H. Area of 'sole horn'

The significance of the lunula is discussed by Burrows (1917). He mentions a number of theories but believes the pale colour is due to looseness of the nail in this region owing to the curious distribution of fibrous tissue beneath it. This, however, is not the whole explanation because the area of the lunula remains visible on the nail plate after avulsion of the nail while the appearance still remains visible on the nail bed. Both nail and nail bed must therefore contribute to the appearance. It is probably due to a combination of incomplete keratinisation in the nail plate and looseness of connective tissue in the nail bed (Lewin, 1965).

Blood supply

The nail matrix and nail bed are richly supplied with blood. The arterial supply originates from two main arterial arches lying below the nail plate. The arteries forming these arches are branches of the digital arteries after they reach the pulp space of the terminal phalanx. The two digital arteries form a cruciate anastomosis in the pulp space and from the point of union branches arise and pass dorsally from the palmar space around the thin waist of the distal phalanx (Fig. 1.5). In this area they are in a confined space bounded medially by the bone and laterally by a dense ligament which extends from the ungual process anteriorly to the lateral ligament of the distal interphalangeal joint behind (Flint, 1955). On emerging from the space the artery divides, one branch anastomosing with its fellow of the opposite side to form a distal arcade and the other to form a proximal arcade. The proximal arcade also receives a contribution from the middle segment of the finger as a vessel passing dorsally over the distal interphalangeal joint (Flint, 1955; see Fig. 1.5). This vessel takes part in the formation of a superficial arcade which supplies blood to the skin at the nail base as well as branches to the proximal arcade. This accessory blood supply is probably responsible for allowing the nail to grow normally when the main digital vessels have been obliterated in the pulp space as may occur in scleroderma of the progressive type (Fig. 1.6) or in pulp space infections. A normal arteriogram (Fig. 1.7) shows the plentiful blood supply to the pulp. For comparison, arteriograms depicting spasm (Fig. 1.8) and arterial blockage (Fig. 1.9) are shown.

The capillary blood supply to the tissues around the nail is abundant. Similar to the capillary loop system of the skin, there exists a capillary loop system supplying the whole of the nail fold (Figs. 1.10, 1.11 and 1.12). In a small area beneath the lunula the loop system was ill-defined in specimens examined by the author, but this may have been the result of incomplete filling (Samman, 1959).

The nail bed is also richly supplied with glomus bodies which are probably concerned in the regulation of the blood supply to the extremities in cold weather. There is also a very rich supply of lymphatic vessels.

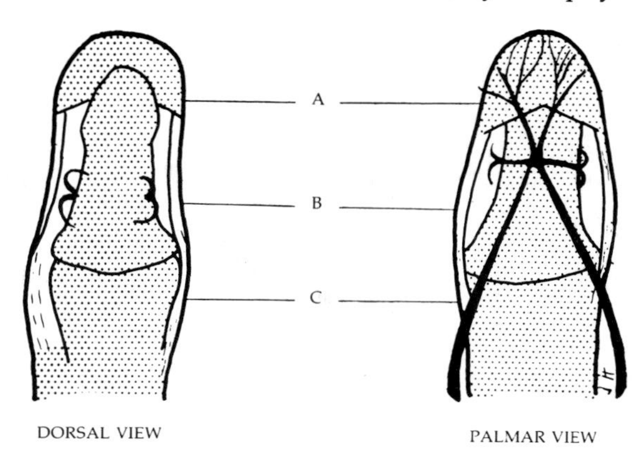

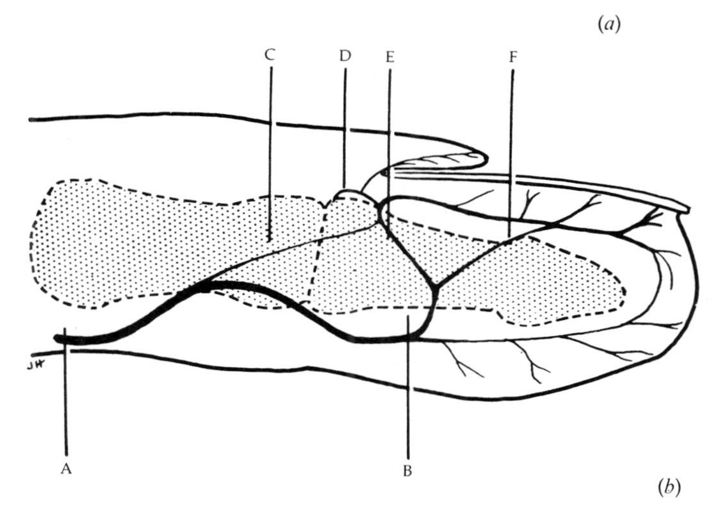

Fig. 1.5 (a) Diagram of main arterial blood supply to the nail bed from above and below. Based on Flint (1955)

A. Ungual spine
B. Interosseous ligament
C. Collateral ligament

(*b*) Diagram of main arterial supply to the nail and nail bed—lateral view. Based on Flint (1955)

A. Digital artery
B. Branch of digital artery arising in pulp space
C. Branch of digital artery arising in middle segment of finger and reaching nail area without passing through pulp space
D. Superficial arcade
E. Subdivision of B to form proximal arcade
F. Subdivision of B to form distal arcade

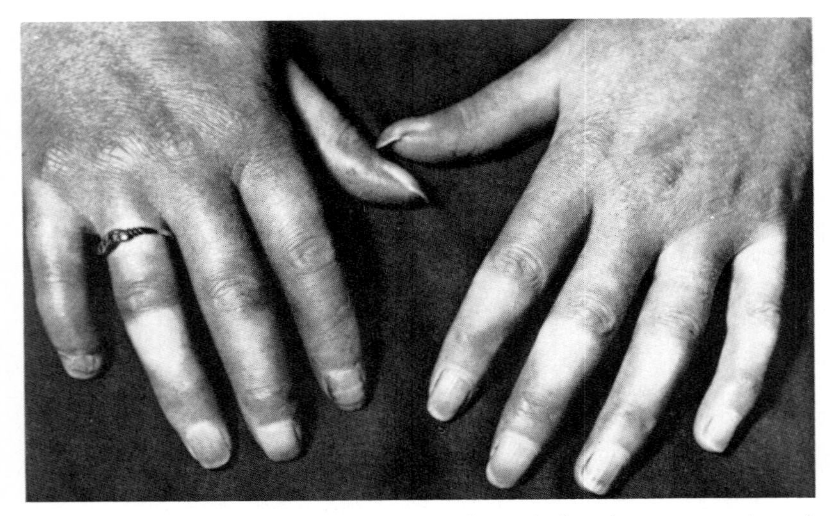

Fig. 1.6 Progressive scleroderma (acrosclerosis) showing preservation of thumb nails in the presence of pulp atrophy. Partial destruction of nail of right little finger

Although the normal blood supply to the nail is so good, defective peripheral circulation is one of the major causes of nail deformities. This is probably largely due to the ease with which the digital arteries go into spasm.

Nail growth

Unlike hairs, nail growth is continuous throughout life and ceases at death. The apparent continuing growth for 2 or 3 days after death is probably due to shrinkage of the soft tissues around the nail. Although the rate of growth varies greatly from person to person, it is fairly constant in any one individual, but is rather more rapid in youth than in old age. This is well shown by Hamilton, Terada and Mestler (1955) who also show that the nails gradually thicken with age. The average rate of growth of finger nails varies between 0.5 and 1.2 mm per week (Hillman, 1955). The author has measured the rate of growth in many nail disorders and can confirm this finding. Bean (1980) has recorded personal observations on the growth of his own thumb nail continuously over periods of 10, 20, 25, 30, and 35 years. He noted a decided slowing during

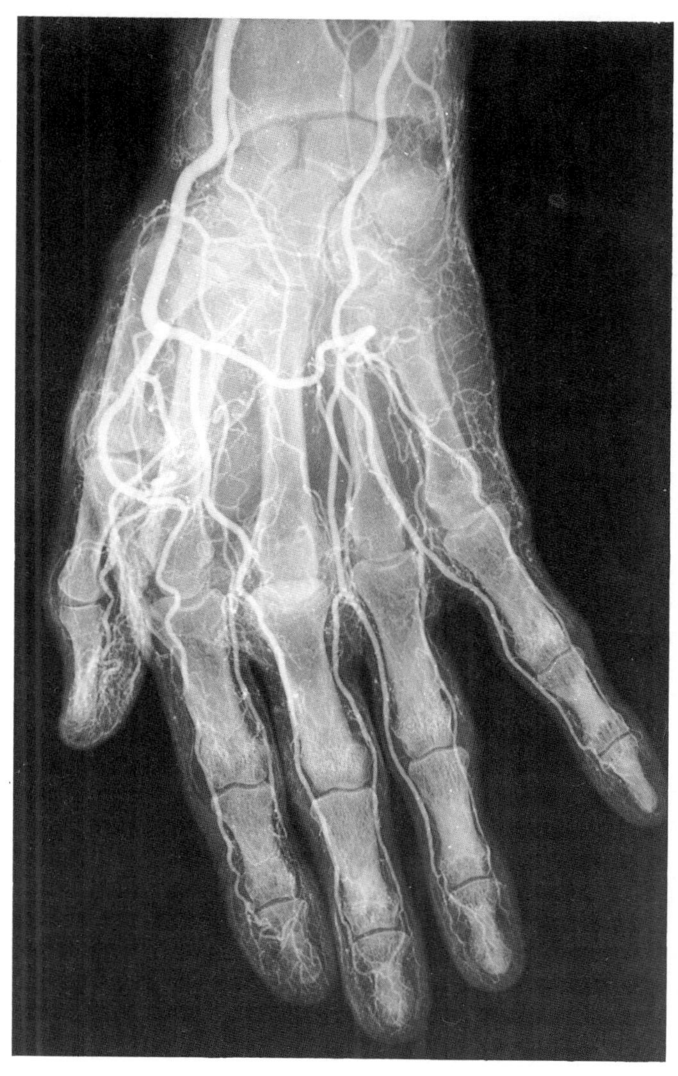

Fig. 1.7 Normal arteriogram of hand

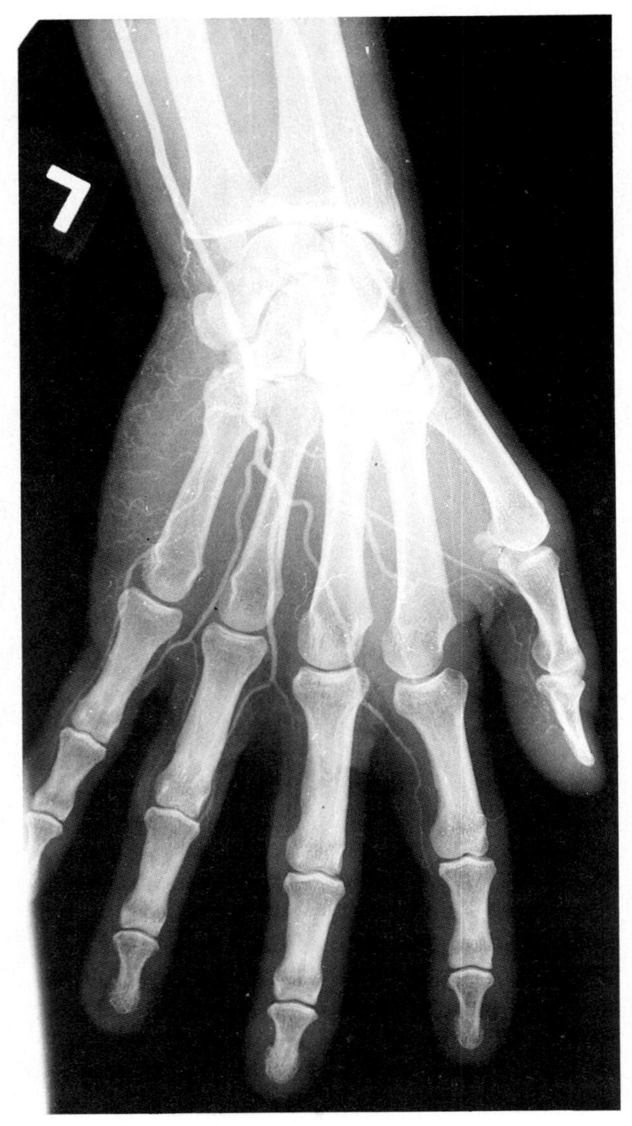

Fig. 1.8 Arteriogram showing spasm of digital vessels

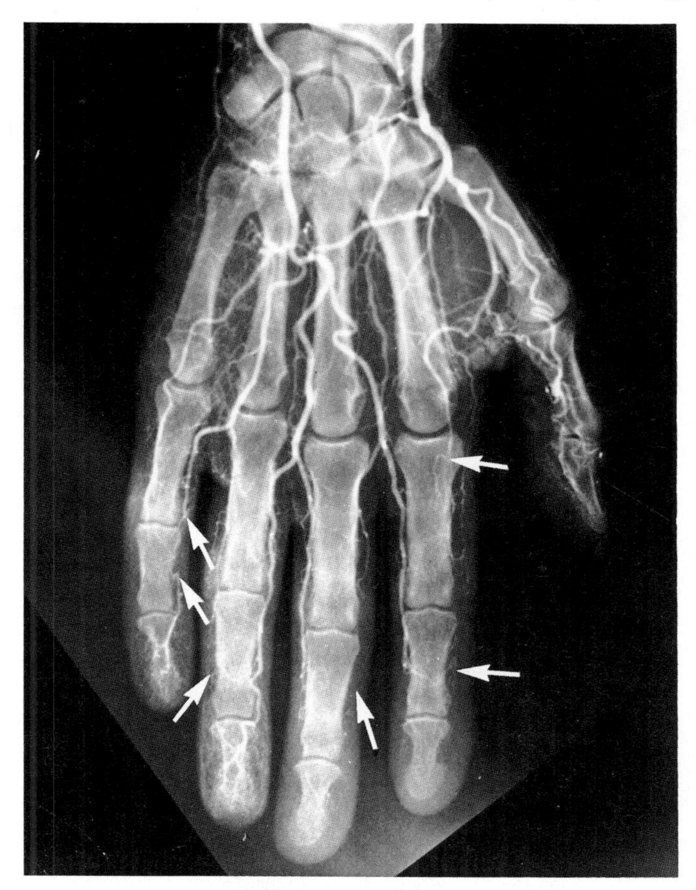

Fig. 1.9 Arteriogram showing organic blockage of many digital vessels

the second period and a levelling out later. Orentreich, Markofsky and Vogelman (1979) took measurements from humans and dogs and showed that there was a reduction in rate of growth of 50% from birth to death. As the life-span of a dog is 20% of a man the rate of decrease was five times greater than in man. In man there are 7-year periods of slow decline alternating with 7-year periods of more rapid decline.

The rate of growth varies slightly from finger to finger as shown by Dawber (1970). This work confirmed the earlier observations of le Gros Clark and Buxton (1938). Generally it may be said that the longer the finger the more rapid the nail

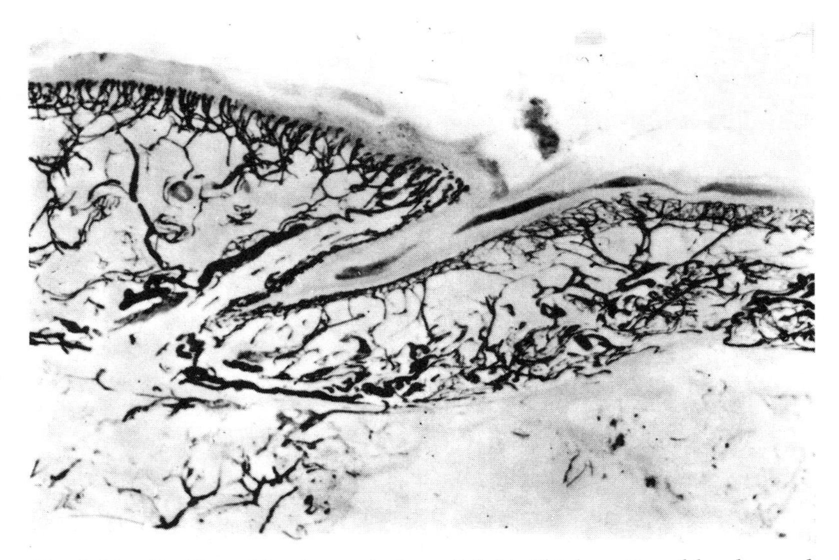

Fig. 1.10 Capillary blood supply to nail fold. Thick section, blood vessels injected anteroposterior

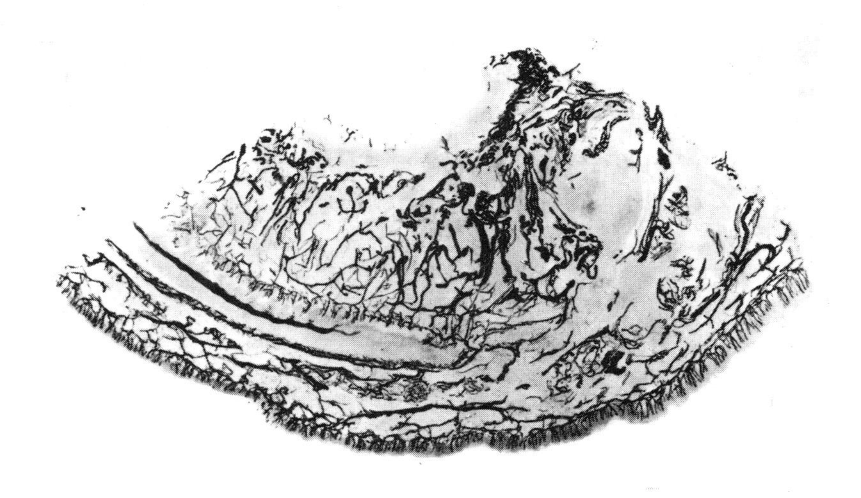

Fig. 1.11 Same as *Fig. 1.10*. Transverse section mid-way between tip of nail fold and cuticle

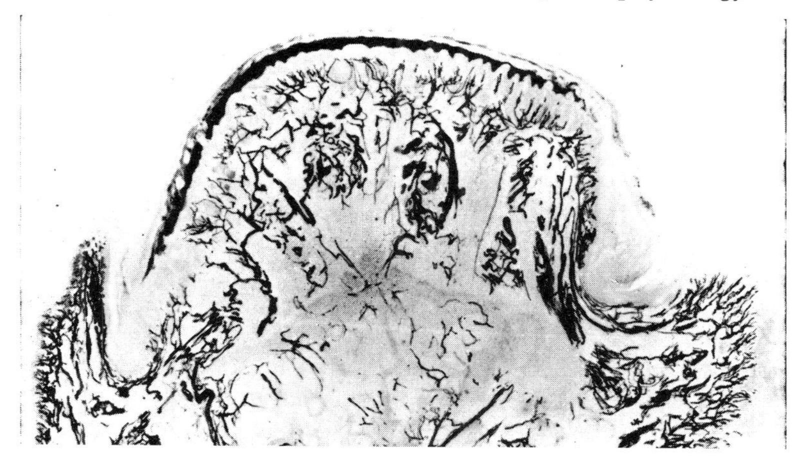

Fig. 1.12 Capillary blood supply to nail bed. Thick section, blood vessels injected—transverse

growth, therefore the middle finger has the most rapid growth followed by index and ring finger, while the thumb and little finger nails have the slowest rate. Nails on the right hand grow slightly quicker than those on the left. Many measurements are required to show up these small but significant differences. Dawber (1970) has also shown that in psoriasis apparently normal nails grow significantly faster (taken as a group) than the corresponding nails of normal subjects. Nails showing pitting grow even faster than the apparently normal nails. Owing to the wide range of normal growth rate, groups of patients rather than individuals have to be considered in these measurements. A similar observation has been made for nails showing idiopathic onycholysis where the rate of growth may be much higher than normal (Dawber, Samman and Bottoms, 1971). Nail growth may also be speeded up in the presence of inflammatory change around the nail and in the bullous form of congenital ichthyosiform erythroderma. Growth rate may be temporarily depressed in many general medical illnesses or generalised skin complaints. Sibinga (1959) observed that measles constantly depressed the rate of nail growth in young children for a short time. Both Bean and Sibinga also noted that a severe attack of mumps caused a temporary slowing of nail growth. Dawber (1981) has shown that nail growth is reduced in a finger which has been immobilised on account of minor injury without nerve injury. He postulates that the reduced growth rate is due to a combination of immobilisation and lack of injury to the finger tip. A bitten nail which is receiving constant trauma grows more rapidly than normal, while a nail freed of all trauma grows more slowly than normal. There is one condition described on p. 126 under the heading of 'yellow nail syndrome' in which the rate of growth is constantly very slow.

The average length of time taken for a finger nail to grow from the matrix to the free edge is about $5\frac{1}{2}$ months. Toe nails grow about a half to one-third of the rate of finger nails and replacement takes 12–18 months. Kligman (1961) wondered why nails should grow forward rather than up, and concluded that it is due to pressure exerted by the posterior nail fold. If a portion of nail matrix is autografted on to skin away from the nail fold it will produce a nail but one which projects straight upwards. Hashimoto *et al.* (1966) believe that forward growth is the result of all matrix cells being orientated in a forward direction.

Structure of nail

Not a great deal of work has been done on the structure of nail, much less than on wool with its great commercial value. The nail plate is curved in both directions (anteroposterior and lateral) giving it greater strength. Light microscopic studies show it to be made up of layers of cells deprived of nuclei and flattened on the plane of the nail surface. Cells in the outermost layer can be examined individually by adhesive tape stripping (Germann, Barran and Plewig, 1980). The individual cells are larger in nails growing more slowly and smaller in nails growing quickly. The normal corneocyte is of irregular polyhedral shape, it is not nucleated and has a distinct but irregular trabecular network.

Forslind (1970) has studied nails with the electronmicroscope and with X-ray diffraction techniques and considers their hardness to be due to the cell arrangement and cell adhesion and the ultrastructural arrangement of keratin fibrils. The latter are intercellular and are mainly orientated parallel to the nail surface from side to side. These findings were confirmed in scanning electronmicroscopic studies (Forslind and Thyresson, 1975). Keratin itself is a protein containing a high proportion of sulphur mainly in the form of cystine and in nail constitutes 9.4% by weight. There is a natural line of cleavage between dorsal and intermediate nails. The dorsal nail is much harder than the intermediate but the latter is more pliable and therefore less brittle. Flexibility of nail depends largely on its water content. During water immersion nail weight increases by 22% over its original weight within 2 hours and then decreases (Finlay *et al.*, 1980). Forslind states that the calcium content of nail is very low and in no case that he studied did it constitute more than 2 parts per 1000 by weight. It is suggested that most of this calcium is in the upper surface of the nail plate and is probably derived from the environment (soap, etc.) rather than from within. Robson and Brooks (1974) studied the distribution of calcium in finger nails from both healthy and malnourished children and found that in kwashiorkor it was not possible to distinguish between dorsal, intermediate or ventral portions in respect of calcium content.

Nitrogen, calcium and a number of other elements in nail were estimated by Veller (1970) in an attempt to assess whether there was any appreciable nutritional loss resulting from the constant growth and clipping of nails. The loss was shown to be negligible.

Harrison and Clemena (1972) have shown that by spark source mass spectrometry it is possible to estimate the quantity of many trace elements in human finger nail clippings.

Using gas liquid chromatography, Greaves and Moll (1976) have estimated the amino acid composition of human nails. Marshall (1980) has shown that there are genetic variations in the protein of human nails. He examined 106 samples of apparently normal nail; 69% showed a characteristic pattern of five high sulphur proteins and three low sulphur proteins. The remainder showed an additional major low sulphur protein. The proportion of nail samples containing the variant was much higher in some families than others.

Walters, Flynn and Marvel (1981) describe a method of measuring the permeability of nail to water, methanol and ethanol which may be of use in formulating topical applications for the treatment of fungal infections.

References

Achten, G (1963) L'Ongle normal et pathologique. *Dermatologica* **126** 229
Achten, G (1972) Histologie ungueale. *Bull. Dell'istituto Derm. S. Gall.* **8** 3
Bean, W B (1980) Nail growth. Thirty five years of observation. *Arch. Intern. Med.* **140** 73
Boas, I (1894) Zur Morphologie der Wirbeltirkralle. *Morphol. Jb. Bd.* **21** 281
Burrows, M T (1917) The significance of the lunula of the nail. *Anat. Rec.* **12** 161
Dawber, R (1970) Finger nail growth in normal and psoriatic subjects. *Brit. J. Derm.* **82** 454
Dawber, R (1981) The effect of immobilisation on finger nail growth. *Clin. Exp. Derm.* **6** 533
Dawber, R, Samman, P D and Bottoms, E (1971) Nail growth in idiopathic and psoriatic onycholysis. *Brit. J. Derm.* **85** 558
Finlay, A Y, Frost, P, Keith, A D and Snipes, W (1980) An assessment of factors influencing flexibility of human finger nails. *Brit. J. Derm.* **103** 357
Flint, M H (1955) Some observations on the vascular supply of the nail bed and terminal segments of the finger. *Brit. J. Plast. Surg.* **8** 186
Forslind, B (1970) Biophysical studies of the normal nail. *Acta Dermvenereol (Stockholm)* **50** 161
Forslind, B and Thyresson, N (1975) On the structure of the normal nail. A scanning electron miscroscope study. *Arch. Derm. Forsch.* **251** 199
Germann, H, Barran, W and Plewig, G (1980) Morphology of corneocytes from human nail. *J. Invest. Derm.* **74** 115
Greaves, M S and Moll, J M H (1976) Amino acid composition of human nail as measured by gas liquid chromatography. *Clin. Chem.* **22** 1608
Hamilton, J B, Terada, H and Mestler, G E (1955) Studies of growth throughout the life span in Japanese; growth and size of nails and their relationship to age, sex, heredity and other factors. *J. Gerontol.* **10** 401
Harrison, W W and Clemena, G G (1972) Survey analysis of trace elements in human finger nails by spark source mass spectrometry. *Clin. Chim. Acta.* **36** 485
Hashimoto, K, Gross, B G, Nelson, R and Lever, W F (1966) The ultrastructure of the skin of human embryos III. The formation of the nail in 16–18 weeks old embryos. *J. Invest. Derm.* **17** 205
Hillman, R W (1955) Finger nail growth in the human subject, rates of growth and variations. *Hum. Biol.* **27** 274
Jarrett, A and Spearman, R I C (1966) Histochemistry of the human nail. *Arch. Derm.* **94** 652
Kligman, A M (1961) Why do nails grow out instead of up? *Arch. Derm.* **84** 313
Le Gros Clark, W E (1959) *The Antecedents of Man*. Edinburgh University Press
Le Gros Clark, W E and Buxton, L H D (1938) Studies in nail growth. *Brit. J. Derm.* **50** 221
Lewin, K (1965) The normal finger nail. *Brit. J. Derm.* **77** 421

Lewin, K, De Wit, S and Ferrington, R A (1972) Pathology of the finger nail in psoriasis. *Brit. J. Derm.* **86** 555

Lewis, B L (1954) Microscopic studies of foetal and mature nail and surrounding soft tissue. *Arch. Derm.* **70** 732

Marshall, R C (1980) Genetic variations in the protein of human nail. *J. Invest. Derm.* **75** 264

Norton, L A (1971) Incorporation of the thymidine-methyl H^3 and glycine $2H^3$ in the nail matrix and bed of humans. *J. Invest. Derm.* **56** 61

Orentreich, N, Markofsky, J and Vogelman, J H (1979) The effect of aging on the rate of linear nail growth. *J. Invest. Derm.* **73** 126

Pinkus, F (1927) Der Nagel. In *Handbuck der Haut und Geschlechtskrankeiten,* ed Jadassohn, J, 1/1 pp. 267–289: Julius Springer, Berlin

Robson, J R K and Brooks, G J (1974) The distribution of calcium in finger nails from healthy and malnourished children. *Clin. Chim. Acta.* **55** 255

Samman, P D (1959) The human toe nail. Its genesis and blood supply. *Brit. J. Derm.* **71** 296

Sibinga, M S (1959) Observations on growth of finger nails in health and disease. *Pediatrics* **24** 225

Terry, R B (1955) The onychodermal band in health and disease. *Lancet* **1** 179

Veller, O D (1970) Composition of human nail substance. *Amer. J. Clin. Nutr.* **23** 1272

Walters, K A, Flynn, G L and Marvel, J R (1981) Physiochemical characterisation of human nail: 1. Pressure sealed apparatus for measuring nail plate permeabilities. *J. Invest. Derm.* **76** 76

Zaias, N (1963) Embryology of the human nail. *Arch. Derm.* **87** 37

Zaias, N and Alvarez, J (1968) The formation of the primate nail plate. An autoradiographic study in the squirrel monkey. *J. Invest. Derm.* **57** 120

2

Principal nail symptoms

P. D. Samman

This chapter is inserted as an aid to diagnosis. The nails can react in relatively few ways, so the same symptoms occur in several different conditions.

The pathological processes responsible for most nail changes are at present unknown; but this should soon be overcome when more nail biopsies are undertaken using newer techniques. Zaias (1967) has described a method of taking longitudinal biopsies through the nail which he claims does not leave a permanent split in the nail. With Alvarez (1967) he described a method of processing a nail biopsy for section. Achten (1972) showed that histological examination of nail clippings may be helpful. The various methods used in nail biopsy are described in Chapter 13 (p. 209).

Absence of nail

Anonychia—absence of the nail from birth—is considered in Chapter 12, p. 191. It may also occur in the nail patella syndrome, p. 187.

Brittleness

Brittle nails are very common, but little is known of the basic pathology. Causes may be local or general. Of the systemic causes impaired peripheral circulation (p. 120) and iron deficiency anaemia are the most frequent, among local causes constant immersion of the hands in water may cause the condition especially if an alkaline is the chief offender (Silver and Chiego, 1940). Diffuse alopecia associated with brittle nails has been recorded as a manifestation of an enzyme disturbance of arginine metabolism (Shelley and Rawnsley, 1956). In many cases the cause is quite obscure. The treatment of brittle nails is considered on p. 107.

Discoloration (Fig. 2.1)

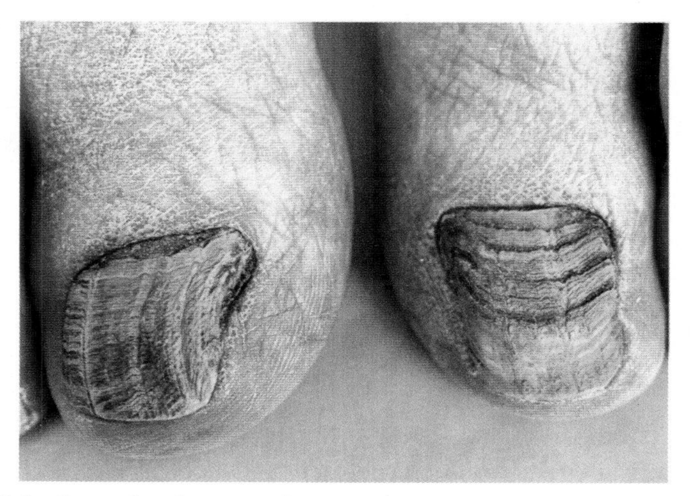

Fig. 2.1 Gross discoloration of great toe nails—possible causes: recurrent subungual haemorrhages; fungal infections; malalignment; other causes see p. 120

The colour of the nail may be altered in many ways and these may be grouped as shown below.

(1) *Staining from external causes:* (Fig. 2.2) dyes encountered at work or in other ways including hair dyes, nicotine, medicaments applied by the patient to himself or others (mercury, vioform, dithranol, resorcin, picric acid, etc.) and tints leaking out of nail varnish (p. 140). *Pseudomonas aeruginosa* infection under or adjacent to the nail will stain the nail black or blue.

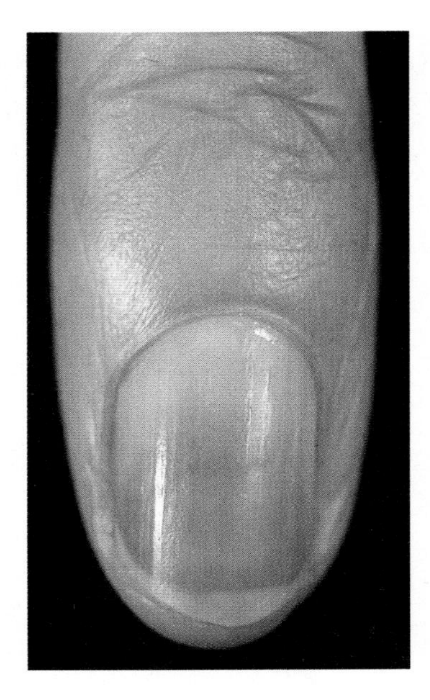

Fig. 2.2 Staining from handling phenol

(2) *Abnormal formation of the nail:* severe psoriasis is the most important condition under this heading. Much less common are acrodermatitis continua, pityriasis rubra pilaris, pachyonychia congenita, alopecia areata and Darier's disease.

(3) *Degenerative changes occurring in a nail after formation:* yellow nail syndrome, congenital ectodermal defect and in old age—all due to the slow growth of the nail.

(4) *Partial destruction after formation:* (Fig. 2.3) fungal and candidal infections often cause a brownish discoloration of the nail but occasionally whiten the nail. Brown or black discoloration of the nail edge is common in chronic paronychia.

(5) *Incorporation of a stain in the nail during formation:* a yellow colour may develop in all nails during prolonged tetracycline administration.

(6) *Miscellaneous causes:* drugs may alter the colour of the nails in other ways (p. 132). In negroid races black streaks are very common and are of little or no significance (p. 177) (Fig. 2.4). A single black streak in a white person may be due to a junctional naevus in the nail matrix (p. 176) (Fig. 2.5); multiple

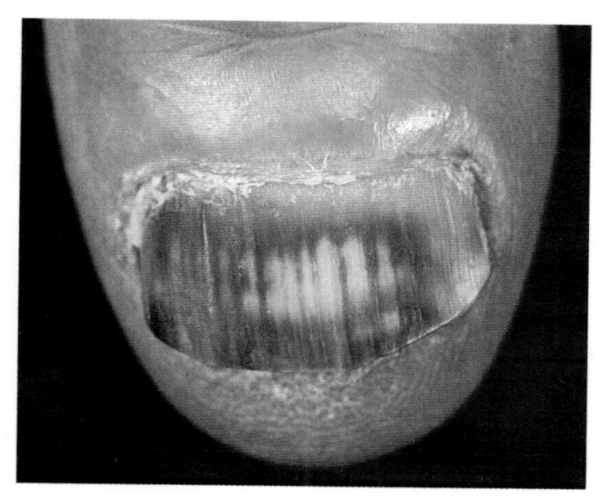

Fig. 2.3 Nail destruction due to fungal infection

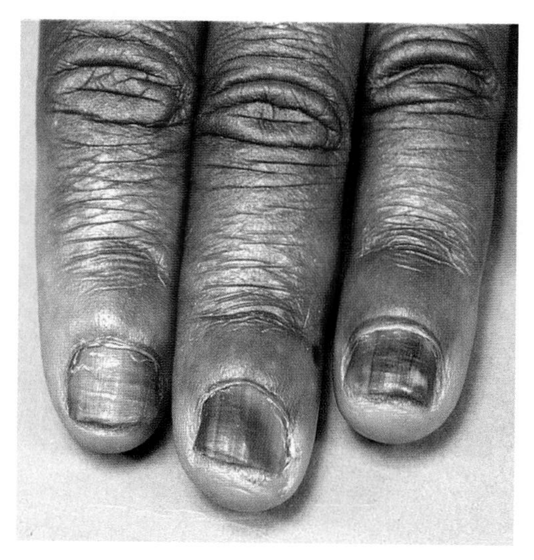

Fig. 2.4 Racial melanonychia

pigment streaks may occur in Addison's disease (Allenby and Snell, 1966). Subcutaneous haemorrhage is the commonest cause of blackening of part of a nail. The half moons may become blue in Kinnier Wilson's disease or red in cardiac failure.

(7) *Leukonychia and whitening* due to changes in the nail bed are considered on pp. 101 and 117.

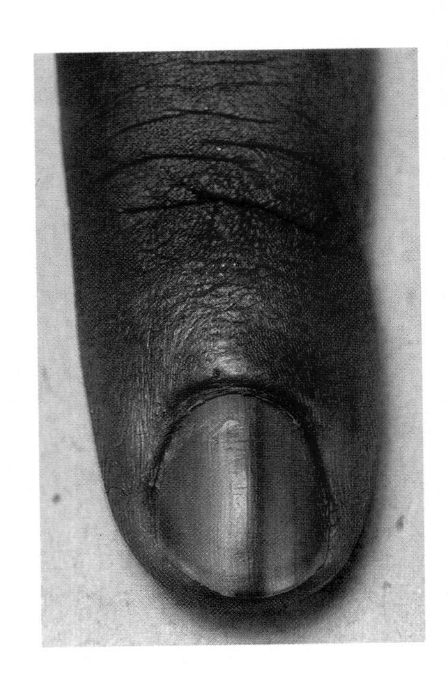

Fig. 2.5 Nail matrix junctional naevus

Lunula abnormalities

Mottling of the lunula may occur in alopecia areata or psoriasis. Triangular lunula may be found in the nail patella syndrome. Colour changes are noted above.

Haemorrhage

Subungual haematomata are almost always due to trauma. Splinter haemorrhages below the nails are discussed on p. 117. In addition to general medical disorders they are also found in psoriasis, dermatitis and fungal infections.

Hypertrophy

Probably the great majority of hypertrophied nails are the result of trauma but they also occur as developmental anomalies in pachyonychia congenita and ectodermal defects. The little toe nail is often thickened as an isolated phenomenon and closely resembles a claw. Sometimes this change is associated with hyperkeratosis of the feet or elsewhere. Touraine and Soulignac (1937) described a case where all toe nails were thickened in association with other developmental anomalies. Stauffer and Simmons (1942) described a number of cases of thickening of the great toe nails. These might be shed and replaced by a nail which again hypertrophied. Some patients also had sebaceous cysts.

Other causes of nail hypertrophy are psoriasis, fungal infections (Fig. 2.6), pityriasis rubra pilaris and Darier's disease.

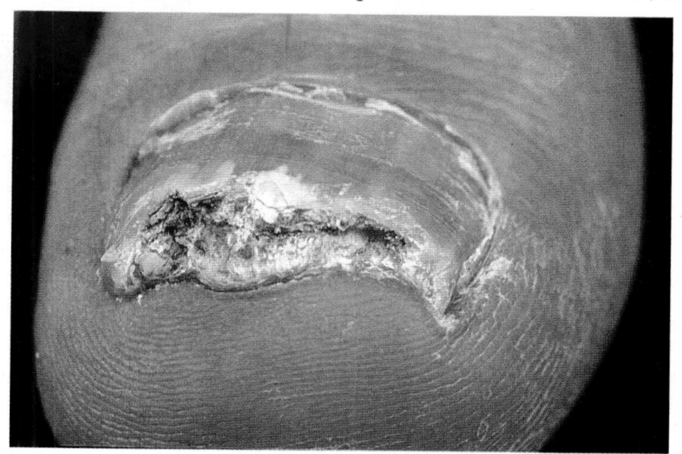

Fig. 2.6 Nail hypertrophy due to fungal infection

Koilonychia

Most characteristically seen as a symptom of iron deficiency anaemia, koilonychia is also found as a congenital anomaly, as a temporary disorder in young children, and in association with thinning of the nail plate from any cause. Both halves of a split nail in the nail patella syndrome may show koilonychia. In some cases no cause can be found.

Onycholysis

Onycholysis—separation of the nail from its bed—is one of the commonest of nail symptoms (Fig. 2.7). It is found as part of

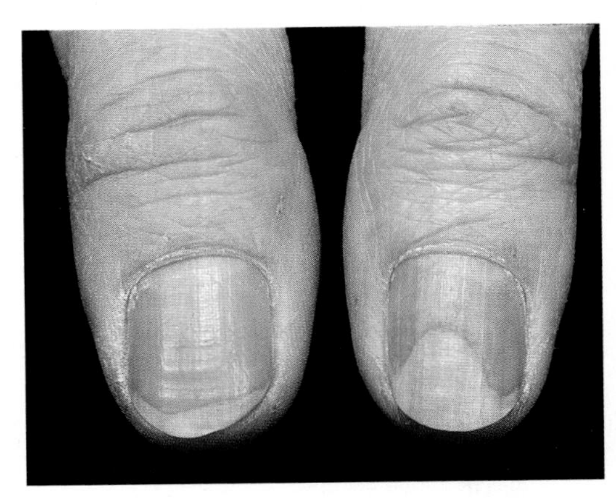

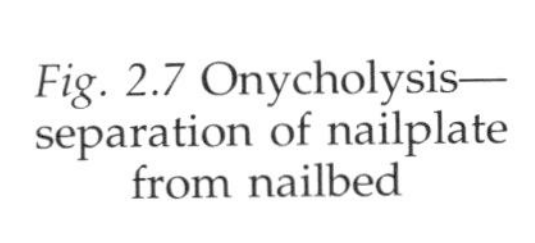

Fig. 2.7 Onycholysis—separation of nailplate from nailbed

the symptomatology of psoriasis, fungal infections, dermatitis of the finger tips and rarely in drug eruptions. It is also found in defective peripheral circulation, the yellow nail syndrome, shell nail syndrome, congenital ectodermal defect, in thyroid disorders and in association with hyperhidrosis. Trauma of various kinds may initiate or aggravate the condition but some cases appear to be idiopathic and these are discussed on p. 97. It is occasionally met with as an occupational disease, for example in poultry pluckers (Forck and Kastner, 1967).

Pitting

Psoriasis is the commonest cause of nail pitting (Fig. 2.8) but pits are also found in dermatitis, alopecia areata (Fig. 2.9) and

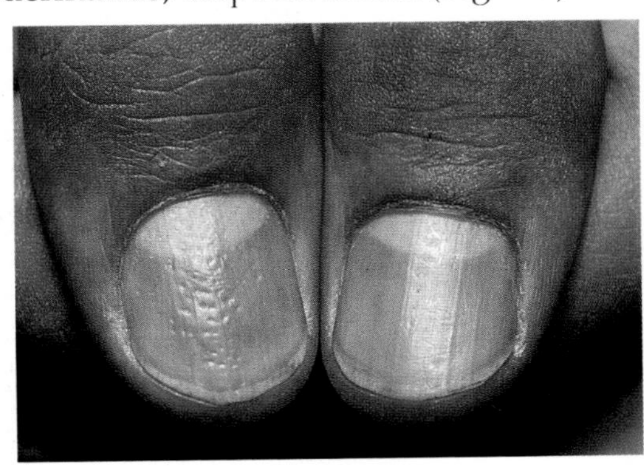

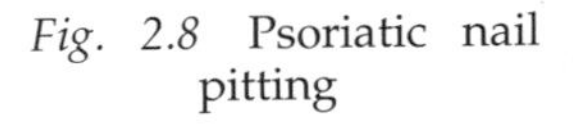

Fig. 2.8 Psoriatic nail pitting

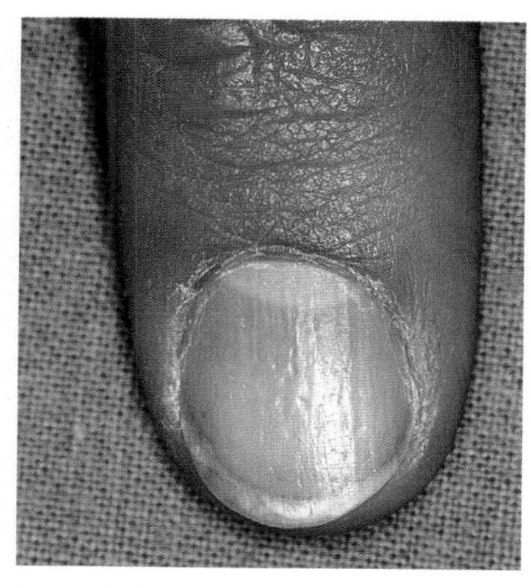

Fig. 2.9 Superficial pits in alopecia areata

fungal infection. Minor degrees of pitting are common in persons with otherwise healthy nails and with no other skin complaints.

Pterygium formation

This is a progressive complaint usually starting on one nail and extending to others (Fig. 2.10). The cuticle appears to grow forward on the nail plate and the nail is split into two

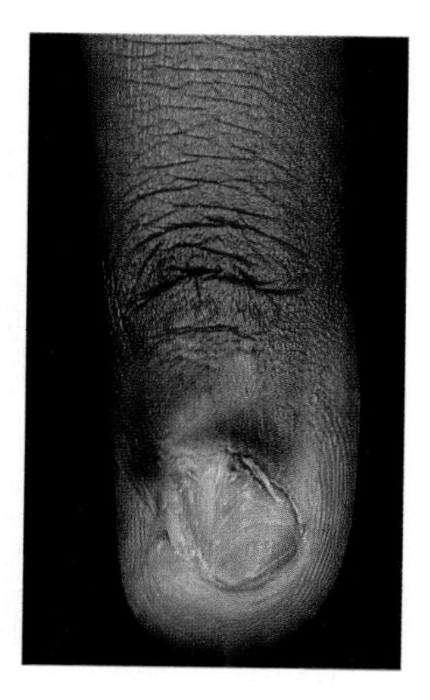

Fig. 2.10 Pterygium formation

portions which gradually get smaller as the pterygium widens. It may extend to complete loss of the nail or small remnants may remain. Histologically it can be seen to result from fusion of the epidermis of the dorsal nail fold to the nail bed including the matrix. It occurs as a result of impaired peripheral circulation and in severe lichen planus. In a few cases, however, no cause can be found including those occurring in idiopathic atrophy of the nail (p. 105).

Shedding

Nail loss may be the result of loosening at the base (onychomadesis) or separation from the nail bed (onycholysis) extending until the whole nail becomes loose and comes away completely. Nail loss should further be divided into loss without and loss with scarring.

Loss without scarring

Periodic shedding is an uncommon congenital anomaly discussed on p. 197. Loss of one or two nails especially the great toe nails is not uncommon and although no cause can normally be found it is probably due to minor trauma in most cases. The nail will often be shed following a subungual haematoma. Severe onycholysis from any cause may progress to temporary nail loss. This is especially characteristic of the yellow nail syndrome (p. 126). The nails are occasionally shed after severe illness (see under Beau's lines p. 115) or as a reaction to drugs (p. 132).

Loss with scarring

This is the most serious nail symptom. It may occasionally follow trauma, defective peripheral circulation, lichen planus, epidermolysis bullosa and bullous drug eruptions. It may occur as part of some congenital anomalies and may be the result of pterygium formation. Although scarring is present, small portions of nail may remain or regrow.

Splitting

Splitting into layers is discussed on p. 160. Splitting longitudinally may be the result of trauma and may be temporary or permanent. Excessively ridged nails (see below) are liable to split along the ridges, as are thin and brittle nails. Some affected nails in the nail patella syndrome may show a single longitudinal split (p. 188).

Striations

Longitudinal striations are common in healthy conditions but are usually of minor degree in young persons, becoming more prominent in old age. Exaggeration of the striations may occur in lichen planus (Fig. 2.11), in Darier's disease, in association with defective peripheral circulation and as a developmental anomaly. They are also said to occur more often in

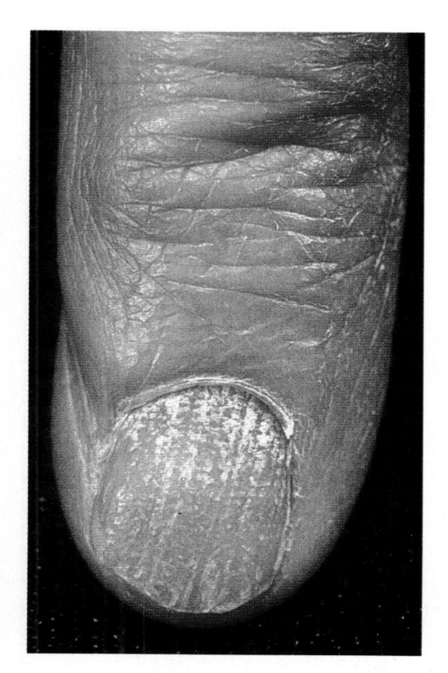

Fig. 2.11 Suggested longitudinal striations (onychorrhexis) in lichen planus

patients with rheumatoid arthritis than normal subjects when the striations may be accompanied by beading.

A single depression through the length of the nail may be due to median dystrophy (p. 99), habit tic (p. 155), or a mucous cyst (p. 174).

Transverse striations of minor degree, and regular in appearance, may occur as a developmental anomaly and they have also been attributed to difference in the rate of growth of the nail at or near the menstrual period compared with at other times. Gross irregular cross-striations are found in dermatitis (Fig. 2.12), and also occur as a result of trauma from excess manicuring or a habit tic. A single depression across a nail may be a Beau's line (p. 115) (Fig. 2.13).

Thinning

Thinning of the nail plate is seen in association with defective peripheral circulation, lichen planus, epidermolysis bullosa and iron deficiency anaemia. In many cases, however, no cause is apparent.

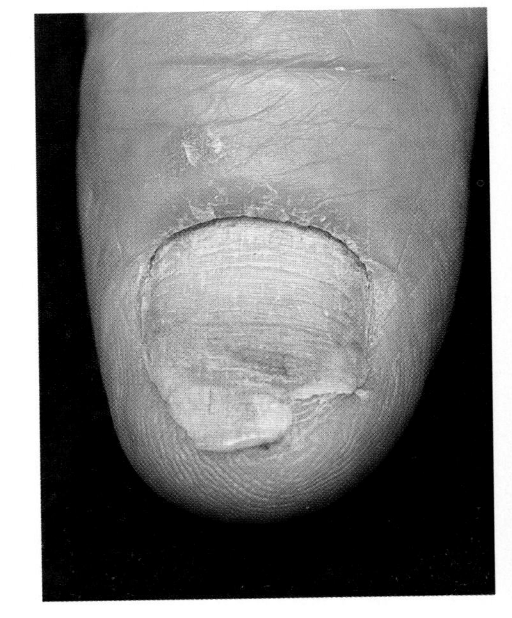

Fig. 2.12 Transverse striations due to dermatitis

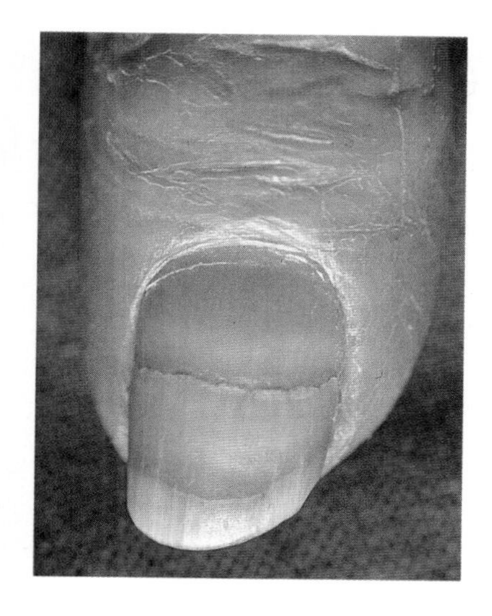

Fig. 2.13 Transverse striations (Beau's line)

References

Achten, G (1972) Histologie ungueale. *Bull. Dell-istuto Derm. S. Gall.* **8** 3

Allenby, C F and Snell, F H (1966) Longitudinal pigmentation of the nails in Addison's disease. *Brit. Med. J.* **1** 1582

Alvarez, R and Zaias, N (1967) A modified polyethylene glycol-pyroxylin embedding method. *J. Invest. Derm.* **49** 409

Forck, G and Kastner, H (1967) Charakteristische Onycholysis Traumatica bei Fliehbandarbeiter in Geflugelschlacterei. *Der Hautarzt* **18** 85

Shelley, W B and Rawnsley, H M (1965) Aminogenic alopecia. Loss of hair associated with argininosuccinic aciduria. *Lancet* **ii** 1327

Silver, H and Chiego, B (1940) Nails and nail changes. Brittleness of nails (fragilitas unguium). *J. Invest. Derm.* **3** 357

Stauffer, J and Simmons, J (1942) Hyperkeratosis of the large toe-nails and sebaceous cysts. *J Hered.* **33** 285

Touraine, A and Soulignac, M (1937) Onychogryphose congénitale généralisée des orteils. *Bull. Soc. Fr. Derm. Syph.* **44** 305

Zaias, N (1967) The longitudinal nail biopsy. *J. Invest. Derm.* **49** 406

3

Infections affecting the nails

R. J. Hay

Nail involvement in the course of an infection may result from direct invasion of the nail apparatus, usually the nail plate or fold, or by encroachment of an infection affecting adjacent structures. In addition to this organisms may colonise spaces beneath the nail plate or folds or invade previously diseased nails. Generally speaking few organisms are capable of invading healthy nail keratin. For instance, only a limited number of fungi, including some dermatophytes, possess enzymes—keratinases—which allow them to utilise the nail plate keratin as an underlying substrate. However, these are amongst the most successful and resistant causes of nail disease.

Onychomycosis (fungal nail infections)

Nail plate invasion in fungal infections usually follows penetration of hyphae along the distal or lateral border on the undersurface of the nail plate (distal and lateral subungual onychomycosis) (Figs. 3.1, 3.2). This is the main route of nail invasion by dermatophytes. Penetration may also originate from the proximal nail fold (proximal subungual onychomycosis) (Fig. 3.3). White superficial onychomycosis differs from the other forms of nail infection as the organisms invade the

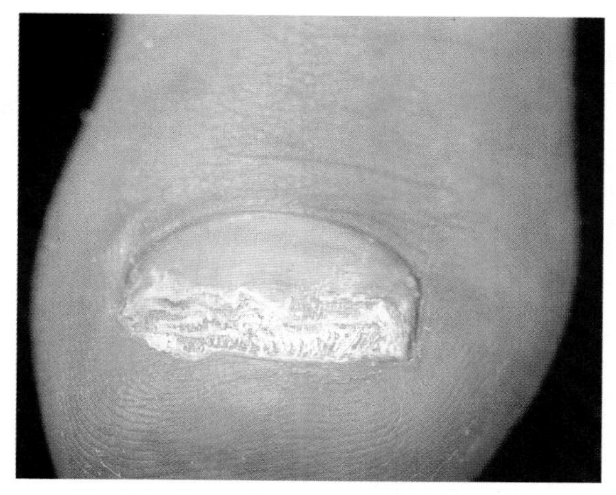

Fig. 3.1 Early fungal infection of toe nail

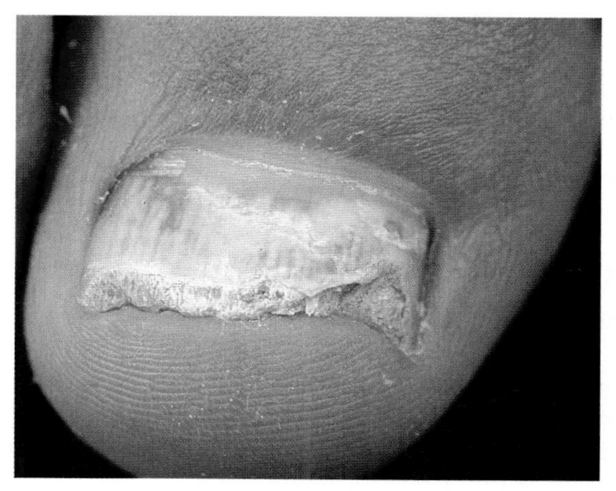

Fig. 3.2 Distal subungual onychomycosis

top surface of the nail. This pattern of onychomycosis may be caused by certain dermatophytes as well as other mould fungi. In this condition the nail plate is covered by discrete or confluent white plaques representing areas of fungal growth. In advanced cases of onychomycosis it is seldom possible to distinguish the original pattern of invasion, as the nail plate may be totally destroyed. In addition to these patterns of primary onychomycosis, fungi may also invade abnormal

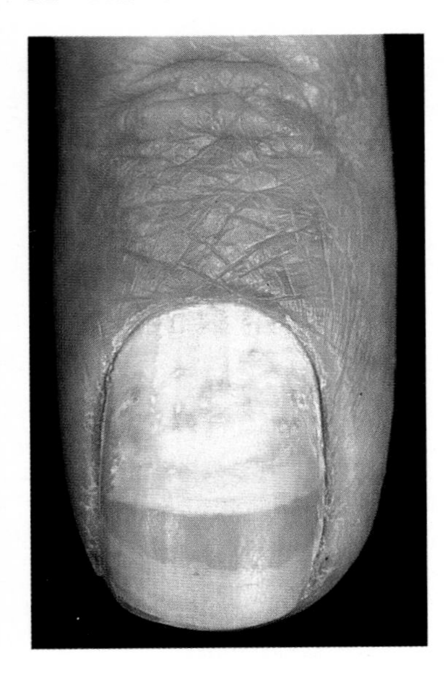

Fig. 3.3 Proximal subungual onychomycosis

nails, for instance candida in onycholytic nails. The main clinical features of onychomycosis caused by different organisms are discussed below (Zaias, 1972).

Onychomycosis due to dermatophytes (tinea unguium)

A number of different dermatophytes may cause nail disease. The commonest are listed in Table 3.1. The usual presenting clinical signs are thickening and opacification of the nail plate along the distal or lateral borders. More rarely there is minimal thickening with onycholysis being the main feature of fungal penetration. The discoloration ranges from white to brown (Figs. 3.4, 3.5). White patches may form following the development of air spaces within the nail plate. The edge of the area of affected nail is usually irregular and often one or more streaks of dystrophic discolored nail extend towards the nail fold from the distal border. Subungual haemorrhages may also occur. In chronic cases the free edge of the nail may become severely eroded with partial or total loss of the nail plate. There may be a residual stump of nail at the proximal

Table 3.1 Dermatophytes causing nail disease

Trichophyton rubrum
T. interdigitale
Epidermophyton floccosum
(*T. schoenleinii, T. violaceum, T. soudanense, T. tonsurans, T. megninii*)

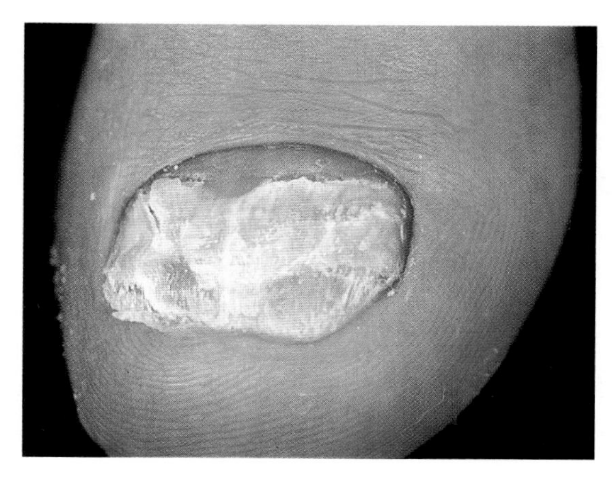

Fig. 3.4 White superficial onychomycosis

nail fold and the underlying nail bed becomes deformed and buckled.

Rarer patterns of dystrophy are seen. Some dermatophytes may cause superficial white onychomycosis (for example, *T. interdigitale*) where the nail is covered by powdery white patches. A similar picture can be seen with *T. rubrum* infections, although it is often accompanied by full thickness nail dystrophy in other areas. Invasion of the proximal nail fold with pain and opacification at the base of the nail is rare. Pitting or ridging of the nail surface may occur in some infections, particularly where the nail is thickened and this is irregularly distributed over the plate. Pits are larger than those seen in psoriasis or alopecia areata. Rarely fungal infections may mimic other nail conditions such as leukonychia striata.

With the exception of the rare instances of onychomycosis caused by dermatophytes in children there is usually evidence of invasion of the skin in the form of interdigital erosion or

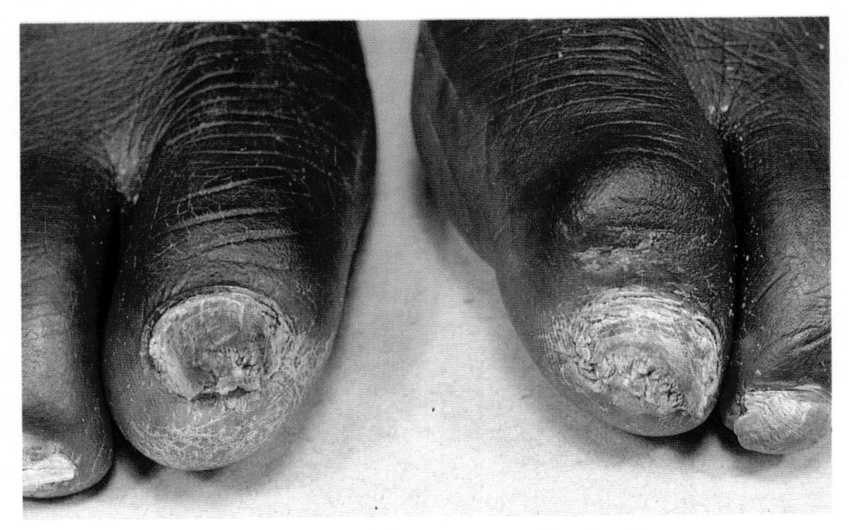

Fig. 3.5 Fungus infection: gross discoloration

scaling of the soles or palms. Where dermatophytes cause finger nail dystrophy they usually involve toe nails as well (compare candida infections). The clinical pattern of unilateral palm scaling and bilateral foot infection is typical of either dermatophytosis or *Hendersonula* or *Scytalidium* infections (see below). Finally, although dermatophytes usually infect healthy nails they may also invade dystrophic nails, particularly after onycholysis (primary or secondary) or onychogryphosis.

Diagnosis

The diagnosis of onychomycosis due to dermatophytes can be confirmed by soaking full-thickness nail clippings in 20% potassium hydroxide. After between 15 and 60 minutes, or longer, the nail becomes soft and can be squashed beneath a cover slip. Sometimes gentle heating is necessary. The cleared nail is examined microscopically with the condenser 'racked down'. Dermatophyte hyphae should be easily visible. The appearances of dermatophyte mycelium in nails are shown in Fig. 3.6 and compared with *Candida* (Fig. 3.7) and *Scopulariopsis* (Fig. 3.8). The appearances are sufficiently dif-

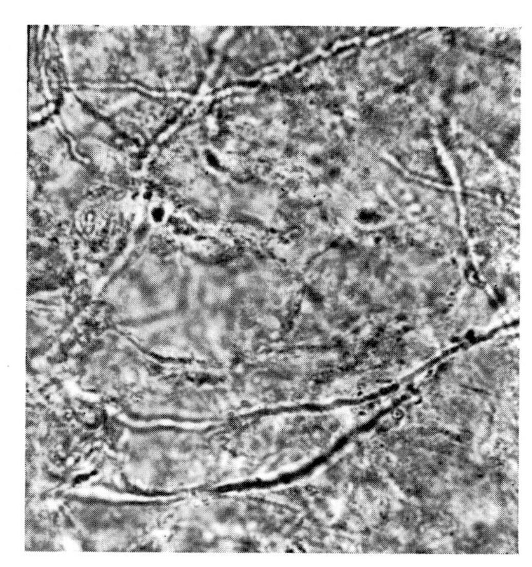

Fig. 3.6 Trichophyton rubrum filaments in potash preparation. Reduced by 50% from × 962

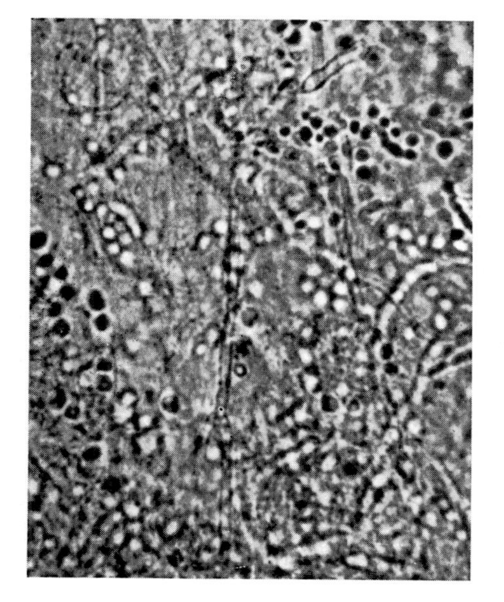

Fig. 3.7 Candida albicans infection of nail plate—potash preparation. (Pseudohyphae and groups of yeasts.) Reduced by 30% from × 612

ferent for the diagnosis to be established with some confidence before the results of culture are available. The viability of dermatophytes in nails is less than from other sites but culture should be attempted using Sabouraud's agar. If specimens are negative at the first attempt the procedure should be

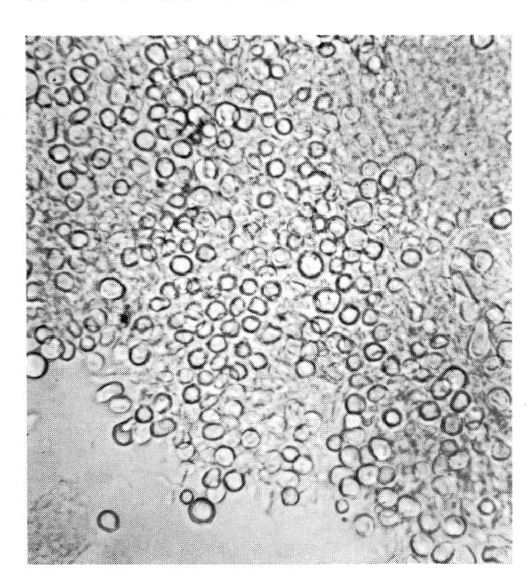

Fig. 3.8 *Scopulariopsis brevicaulis* infection of nail plate—potash preparation (group of large spores, some pear-shaped). Reduced by 50% from × 962

repeated before committing the patient to long-term therapy. Alternative methods of sampling the infected nail include removal of nail material obtained with a dental drill close to the proximal edge of the fungal invasion. It is not uncommon, particularly in the toe nails, to find mixed infections, of dermatophytes and other organisms such as *Hendersonula toruloidea* (p. 45).

Treatment

Onychomycosis caused by dermatophytes seldom responds to topical antifungal therapy because of the deep location of the infection. Although claims of successful treatment have been obtained using topical imidazole (such as econazole) lotions or creams or cyclopyroxolamine, these are very uncommon except in white superficial onychomycosis. In very early infections the new topical nail lacquer containing amorolfine has been reported to produce recoveries in over 50% of patients. For adequate treatment it is usually necessary to treat patients with an oral antifungal such as griseofulvin (Davies, 1980). Griseofulvin is given in a dose of 15 mg/kg daily (usually 1 g daily for an adult with food). Some patients experience the common side-effects of headache and nausea. In these circumstances it is worth reducing the dose by using 125 mg tablets and slowly increasing the daily intake until side-effects are encountered. In this way it is often possible to find a maximum tolerable dose of griseofulvin. It is seldom worth increasing the daily dose of griseofulvin beyond 1.5 g. Progress should be reviewed regularly and the emergence of new uninfected nail at the proximal nail fold should be apparent within 2–3 months. Treatment has to be continued for at least 6–9 months in finger nail infections and 9–18 months for toe nails. It is seldom possible to achieve remission of infections which have not responded after 18 months. Although the remission rate is high (over 80%) in finger nail infections, toe nails respond poorly (Davies, Everall and Hamilton, 1967) particularly in the elderly or patients with predisposing abnormalities such as peripheral vascular disease; the relapse rate is high. It is always advisable to discuss the treatment carefully with the patient before embarking on long-term therapy.

More recently there have been two additions to the antifungal range and, where they are available, they are recommended in place of griseofulvin. Terbinafine and itraconazole offer better long-term results. With terbinafine there are a number of studies showing that treatment for 6 weeks for finger nails and 12 weeks for toe nails is often sufficient to produce long-term recoveries in over 70–80% of those on treatment (Goodfield, 1992). With itraconazole an increased dose of 200 mg may prove to be similarly effective in both finger and toe nail infections given over 12 weeks (Willemsen *et al.*, 1992). The use of intermittent regimens using one week's therapy per month is also being investigated. There is little data on the use of fluconazole in onychomycosis at present. The role of ketoconazole, which may sometimes cause hepatatis (Heiberg and Svejgaard, 1981) in this condition has largely been superseded in many countries by itraconazole or terbinafine. Toxicity data for both terbinafine and itraconazole indicates that nausea, gastrointestinal discomfort and headache are uncommon. Reports of more serious adverse effects such as liver injury are extremely rare with either drug.

Alternative methods of managing onychomycosis due to dermatophytes include partial or total nail removal or chemical ablation using 40% urea paste. The latter is applied to the affected plate under an impermeable occlusive dressing such as cellophane, the whole area being carefully bandaged. Treated nails should be exposed after 1 or 2 weeks, the softened nail can be cut away and the nail bed lightly curetted. Patients should receive topical or oral antifungal therapy for at least 2 months after nail removal. The relapse rate is relatively high after nail ablation, and the latter is best reserved for patients who have residual nail involvement after prolonged oral antifungal treatment. There are also complications after nail removal. For instance if infections have been present for a number of years the nail bed becomes heaped and distorted. The regrowing nail may dig into the lateral nail folds leading to secondary infection and ingrowth.

Candida infections

Candida species play an aetiological role in two main forms of nail infection, paronychia (see p. 51) and onychomycosis. In addition, it may merely colonise the undersurface. Nail plate invasion may also follow the development of a candida paronychia. There is still some disagreement over the precise role candida plays in nail disease in the absence of paronychia and in most instances it is probably a secondary coloniser of abnormal nails. Onycholysis, in particular, appears to be associated with secondary nail invasion. Usually the finger nails alone are infected and there is an underlying disease such as Raynaud's phenomenon or peripheral vascular disease which leads to onycholysis. In these circumstances candida invades the superficial aspect of the undersurface of the nail along the distal and lateral borders thus accentuating the onycholysis. While it may be difficult, even with careful direct microscopy, to decide whether candida is colonising a dystrophic nail or contributing to nail dystrophy, the response to ketoconazole or itraconazole therapy in such cases has convinced many observers that the organism is behaving as a secondary pathogen. In patients with Cushing's syndrome candida may cause severe nail dystrophy with distal erosion of the plate. In chronic mucocutaneous candidosis nail plate invasion, opacification and thickening leading to partial or total loss of the nail, often in the absence of paronychia, are diagnostic features. In conclusion it appears that *Candida* species, nearly always *C. albicans*, can cause nail dystrophy, although in most instances they are secondary invaders of abnormal nails (Hay and Clayton, 1982).

The commonest form of nail dystrophy associated with candida is invasion of the lateral finger nail plate secondary to paronychia (Fig. 3.9). The free margin of the nail shows onycholysis and becomes opaque, often with a yellowish or green discoloration. Extension of the infection laterally across the nail surface is rare unless the patient has some form of peripheral vascular disease.

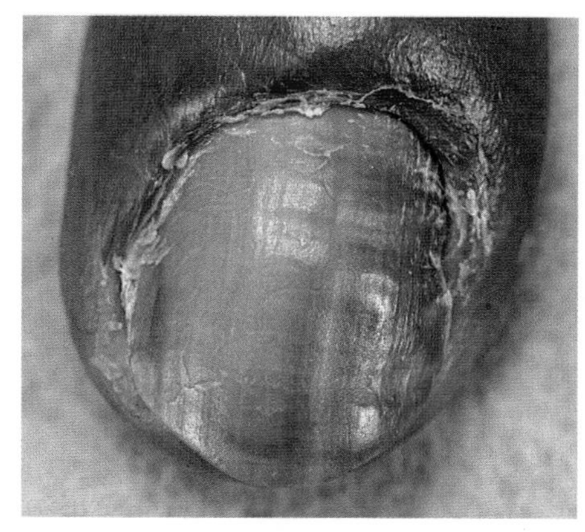

Fig. 3.9 Chronic paronychia: discoloration of edges of affected nails

Invasion of the distal or lateral border of the finger nail may also occur in the absence of paronychia, usually in patients with peripheral vascular disease or Raynaud's syndrome (Fig. 3.10). Onycholysis is usually confined to a narrow strip at the lateral edge but may extend from the distal edge of the nail for some distance beneath the nail plate (Fig. 3.11). The border of the area of onycholysis is usually clearly defined without the wavy contour often seen in psoriasis. Nail thickening is rare and the affected nail is opaque and yellowish in colour. Some patients report pain from the area. More extensive nail invasion with partial loss and ridging of the plate may also occur, particularly in patients with Cushing's syndrome.

In chronic mucocutaneous candidosis any part of the nail apparatus, including the fold, may be affected. Onycholysis and opacification are common but, in addition, considerable hyperkeratosis may develop leading to loss of the nail plate, and obliteration of the normal architecture of the distal finger (Fig. 3.12). Toe nails are only rarely infected by candida. There

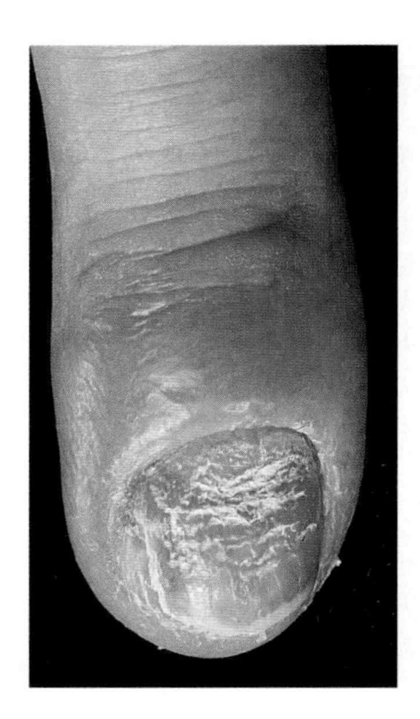

Fig. 3.10 Candida albicans infection of nail plate in patient with Raynaud's syndrome

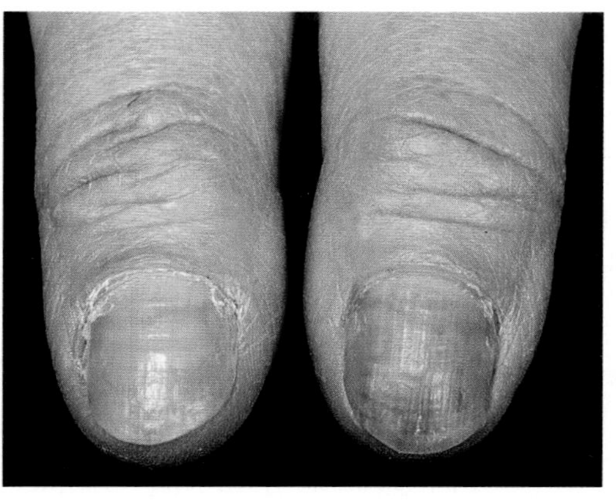

Fig. 3.11 Onycholysis with candida infection

is also no involvement of palms or soles unless there is a concurrent dermatophyte infection.

Diagnosis

The diagnosis of candida infection of the nails can be confirmed in the laboratory by examining nail clippings by

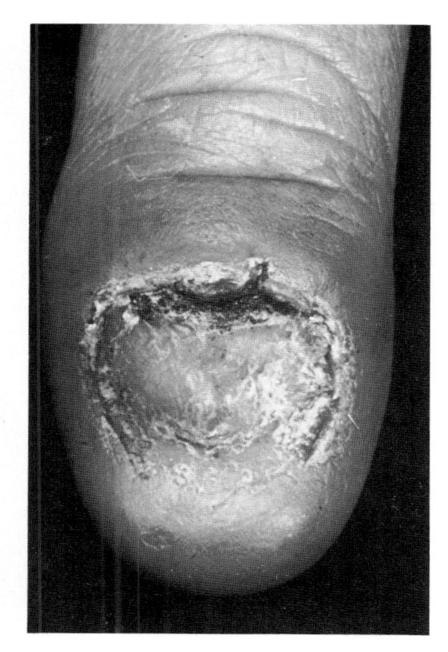

Fig. 3.12 Nail destruction in mucocutaneous candidosis

direct microscopy and by culture. The presence of yeasts and hyphae in nails is diagnostic. The isolation of species of *Candida* other than *C. albicans* should be treated with caution as they rarely contribute to nail disease other than paronychia.

Treatment

True nail plate invasion caused by *Candida* is best treated with oral therapy such as itraconazole (100–200 mg daily) or ketoconazole (200 mg daily), or chemical removal followed by local antifungal treatment, although some preliminary data with amorolfine suggest that this agent may be effective in some cases (Reinel, 1992). If ketoconazole is used, patients should be carefully monitored for hepatic reactions with regular liver function test assessments. The duration of oral therapy is variable but remissions in finger nail infections may take 3–6 months; toe nail infections need longer periods of treatment.

Superficial white onychomycosis

In superficial white onychomycosis the superior aspect of the nail plate is invaded. The affected area of nail is white and crumbly (Zaias, 1966) and it is also usually irregular, although patches may be found on parts of the nail plate in contact with the adjacent digit. Initial lesions are small in discrete patches which tend to coalesce. Eventually they may cover the whole nail surface (Fig. 3.13). The commonest causes are *T. interdigitale, T. rubrum, C. albicans* (in infants), *Acremonium* and *Fusarium* spp.

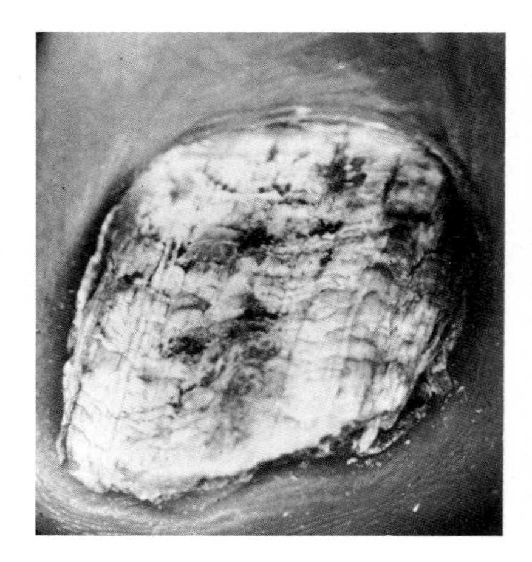

Fig. 3.13 Superficial white onycho mycosis: aspergillus infection

It is relatively easy to obtain material from infected nails for microscopy and culture by gently scraping out white areas. A mass of hyphae or small fragments of mycelium can be demonstrated by direct microscopy.

Affected areas can be treated by topical imidazole antifungal agents twice daily. In recalcitrant cases it may be helpful to scrape out affected areas and treat the nail with topical antifungal agents. If *T. rubrum* is involved the infection may extend deeply through the nail plate and oral antifungal therapy will be necessary.

Onychomycosis due to *Hendersonula toruloidea* and *Scytalidium hyalinum*

Hendersonula toruloidea (Scytalidium dimidiatum) and *Scytalidium hyalinum* are two mould fungi which cause onychomycosis, usually secondary to infection of the skin itself. *H. toruloidea* is a plant pathogen whereas *S. hyalinum* has never been isolated from the natural environment. Although nail infections are typically seen in immigrants from the tropics living in temperate climates, cases are described from the tropics where the condition has been specifically searched for. Endemic areas include the Caribbean, northern South America, East and West Africa, the Indian subcontinent and the Far East.

The nail changes caused by these organisms are indistinguishable and similar to dermatophytosis (Hay and Moore, 1984). Often there is dry scaling of the palms, soles or toe webs. The nail plate is thickened and onycholysis occurs (Fig. 3.14). In some patients the infected nail is hyperpigmented. Characteristic features of nail plate invasion include prominent lateral onycholysis without significant thickening which may spread rapidly and lead to shedding of the nail and, in the finger nails, secondary paronychia. Hyphae on direct microscopy are tortuous and irregular. The organisms grow on Sabouraud's agar but are inhibited by cycloheximide.

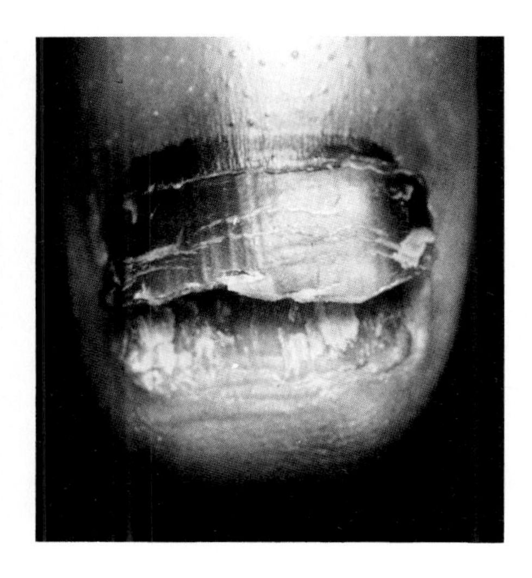

Fig. 3.14 Hendersonula toruloidea infection of nail

Dermatophytes may also be isolated from infected nails. Both *H. toruloidea* and *S. hyalinum* are nail pathogens and their isolation is usually an indication that they are the cause of the nail infection. There is no effective treatment for onychomycosis caused by these fungi.

Onychomycosis due to *Scopulariopsis brevicaulis*

Nail infections caused by *Scopulariopsis brevicaulis* are mainly seen in older patients or those with peripheral vascular disease. The affected nail shows distal or lateral nail plate invasion with a variable degree of thickening and onycholysis. The plate is opaque and characteristically develops a fawn to cinnamon colour (Belsan and Fragner, 1965). The proximal extension of the infection into the nail may show an irregular or scalloped edge (Fig. 3.15). Frequently a single nail (usually the hallux) is infected. Finger nails are not involved but scaling or erosion of the toe webs has been recorded with this organism.

Hyphae present in the nail plate are irregular and may show characteristic thick walled conidia which are hexagonal in shape, lightly pigmented and have a spiny margin.

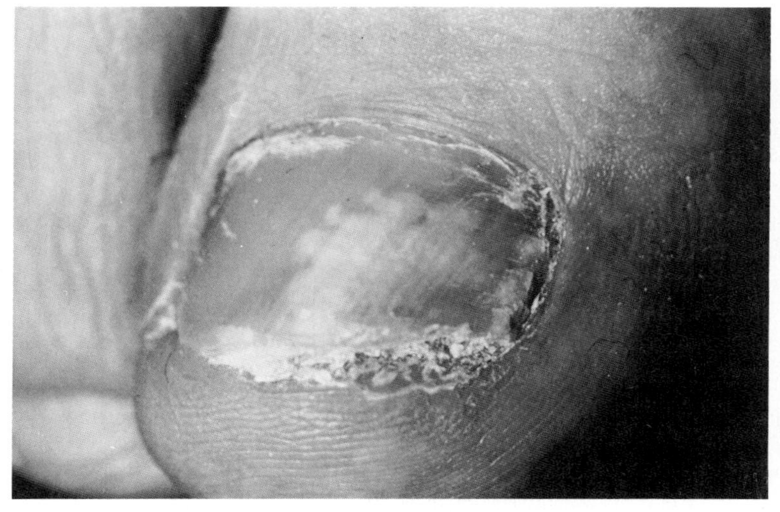

Fig. 3.15 Infection of nail with *Scopulariopsis brevicaulis*

The organism grows on normal media but is inhibited by cycloheximide. *S. brevicaulis* may also be isolated from beneath onycholytic nails or from normal skin and positive cultures should be interpreted carefully. There is no specific treatment but isolated successes may be obtained by using econazole lotion or following chemical (urea) nail ablation.

Onychomycosis due to other fungi

On rare occasions fungi other than those mentioned previously may affect the nails (see Fig. 3.13). These include *Aspergillus terreus, A. versicolor, A. candidus, Acremonium* spp, *Penicillium* spp and *Pyrenochaeta unguium hominis* (English, 1976). The pathogenicity of these organisms remains questionable as they may simply be saprophytes isolated from beneath the nail particularly if there is pre-existing onycholysis. Likewise species of *Candida* other than. *C. albicans,* such as *C. guilliermondii* or *C. parapsilosis,* or other yeasts including *Rhodotorula rubra* may be isolated under similar circumstances (see above). In the case of mould fungi it is usually assumed that they are contributing to the nail dystrophy if structures compatible with the fungi isolated, such as *Aspergillus* fruiting heads, are seen in direct microscopy within nails or if the organisms are isolated repeatedly on at least four occasions. It is also necessary to exclude the presence of another nail pathogen such as a dermatophyte fungus.

Under these circumstances it may be worth attempting to eradicate the fungi, for example with econazole lotion, or to remove the nail plate with 40% urea. None of the non-dermatophyte moulds respond to griseofulvin or ketoconazole. Some, such as *Aspergillus* spp, may respond to itraconazole. However, one must remember that these organisms are invading abnormal nails, for instance, in patients with severe peripheral vascular disease, and the primary disease process needs to be treated if this is possible.

Bacterial infections affecting the nail

A characteristic green discoloration of the nails is seen with heavy colonisation by *Pseudomonas aeruginosa* (Figs. 3.16, 3.17).

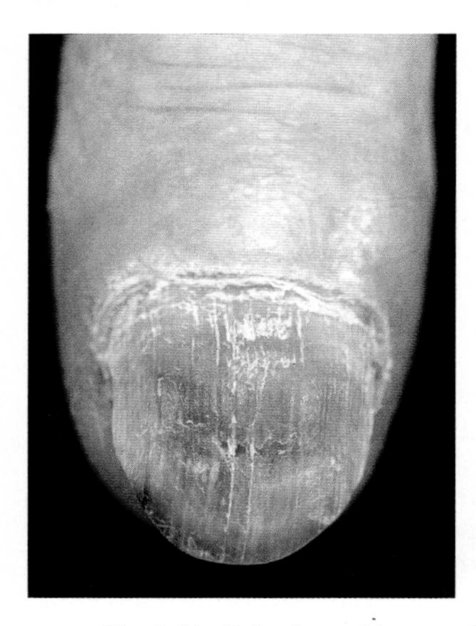

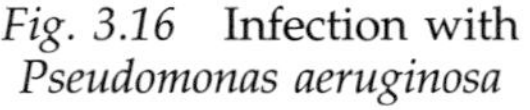

Fig. 3.16 Infection with *Pseudomonas aeruginosa*

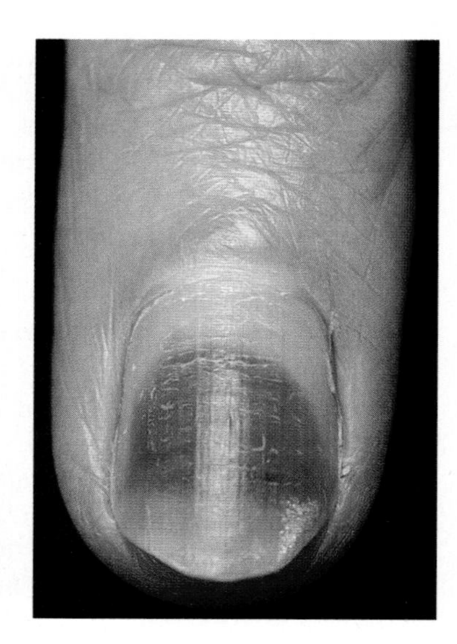

Fig. 3.17 Infection with *Pseudomonas aeruginosa*

This organism can proliferate beneath nails which develop primary or secondary onycholysis. The colour ranges from a dark to a lighter shade of green.

The condition is managed by applying either 1% gentamicin lotion or an antiseptic such as 4% thymol in chloroform beneath the nail. Patients should be instructed to keep affected nails dry and avoid prolonged immersion of unprotected hands in water to prevent recurrences.

Other bacterial infections are uncommon apart from acute bacterial paronychia (p. 51). In primary syphilis a chancre may develop in the fingertip area as a rare manifestation of the disease. Leprosy may lead to traumatic dystrophy with nail plate thickening and ridging through anaesthesia of the digits

Viral infections involving the nails

Primary herpes simplex (HSVI) infections involving the terminal phalanx, herpetic whitlow, may affect the nail (Fig. 3.18). The lesion is often painful and the inflammation may

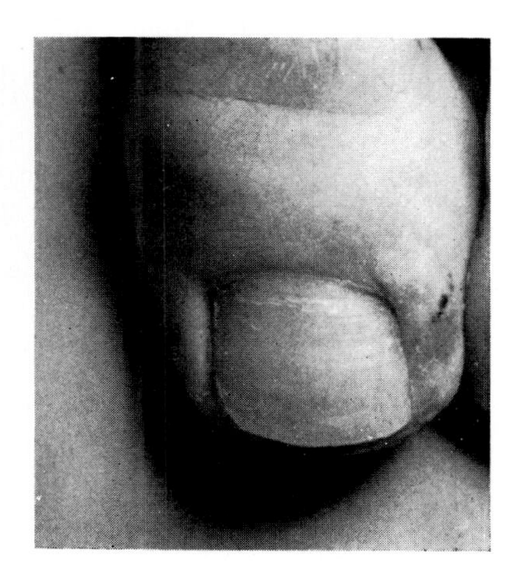

Fig. 3.18 Herpetic whitlow

involve the proximal or lateral nail folds. A small cluster of vesicles can usually be distinguished. The presence of the latter should prevent confusion with acute paronychia. The vesicle fluid is usually clear early in the infection although it may become milky in later stages. The diagnosis can be confirmed by demonstrating the characteristic balloon cells in smears from vesicle fluid. Viral cultures will also confirm the clinical diagnosis. The application of acyclovir 5% cream will shorten the period of infection.

The viral infection, orf, can rarely mimic an acute paronychia although here the primary lesion is usually a large pustule on the finger which occasionally affects the nail folds.

Human papilloma virus infections (common warts) may also affect the proximal and lateral nail fold and cause some buckling of the nail plate by pressure. Periungual warts are often difficult to treat as they may extend under the nail plate for short distances (see also p. 169).

Scabies

In scabies ova of *Sarcoptes scabeii* may be found beneath the nail. This is seen in an extreme form in patients with Norwegian or crusted scabies where the nails may become soft and thickened and may contain large numbers of both ova and acari (Fig. 3.19).

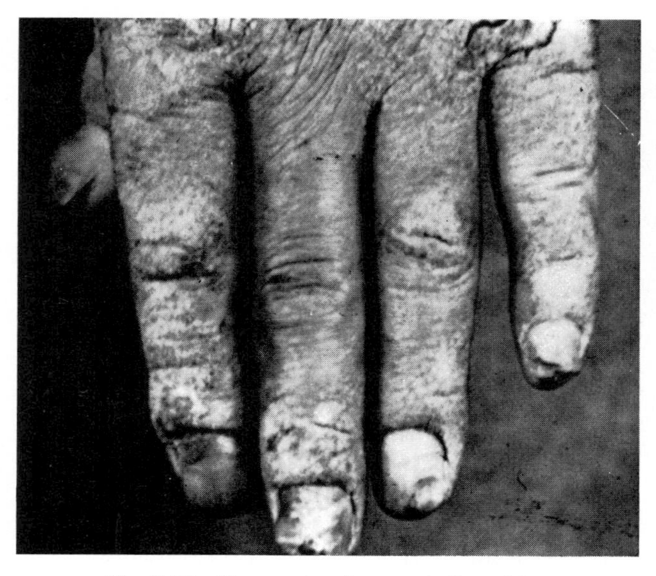

Fig. 3.19 Norwegian (or crusted) scabies

Paronychia

A paronychia is a common inflammatory reaction affecting the nail fold. It may be an acute infection in which pain and the formation of pus are prominent features. The nail is only rarely deformed in acute paronychia. The nail fold becomes tense and red due to localised abscess formation. The latter may subsequently point and granulation tissue may form (Fig. 3.20). This form of infection is usually caused by *Staphylococcus aureus* and only rarely by *C. albicans*. Paronychia may also be chronic. Here the nail fold is swollen and uncomfortable but not exquisitely painful (Fig. 3.21). There is usually loss of cuticle and a clear space between the nail fold and nail plate can be distinguished (Fig. 3.22). Pus can often be expressed from this area by exerting gentle pressure on the nail fold. The formation of pus may follow secondary bacterial infection. In chronic infections the nail plate is often irregular with transverse ridging (Fig. 3.23). Lateral nail plate invasion may develop and the affected nail lesions are yellow or greenish in colour (see Fig. 3.9). Under these circumstances the nail involvement is usually restricted to a narrow strip at the lateral margin. Paronychia are usually confined to finger nails, the commonest digits involved being the index and middle fingers of the right hand and the middle finger of the left. Chronic paronychia are also most commonly seen in women, their development often being associated with repeated exposure to water where cracking of the nail fold skin allows penetration of organisms as well as food and irritant materials such as detergents. The resulting inflammation is therefore multifactorial. Paronychia may also develop in patients with skin disease affecting the nail folds such as eczema, perniosis or psoriasis, or in occupational groups such as bartenders, cooks or laundry workers who have frequent exposure to water. This condition may occur at any age but most patients are between 30 and 60 at the time of onset (Esteves, 1959). Affected men usually develop the condition as a result of their occupation (Frain-Bell, 1957). It is also occasionally seen in children as a result of thumb-sucking (Stone and Mullins, 1968).

In acute cases *S. aureus* is usually isolated. However, in chronic forms of paronychia *Candida* species, particularly *C. albicans* and gram-negative bacteria such as *Proteus* or *Klebsiella* sp may be cultured. Their presence is thought to be secondary to the development of nail fold inflammation, but in turn they may aggravate the condition. Treatment is therefore concerned

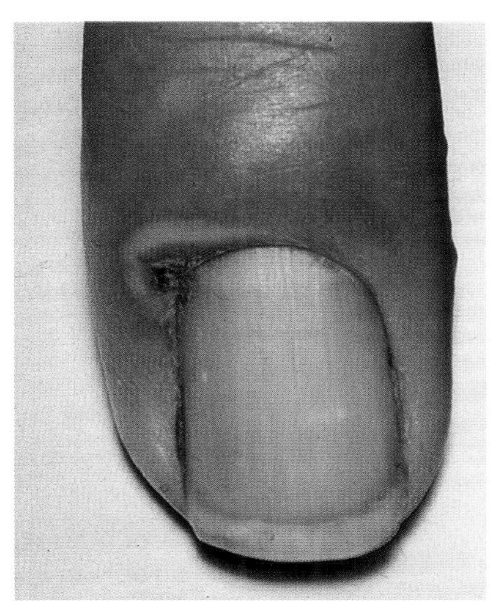

Fig. 3.20 Acute paronychia

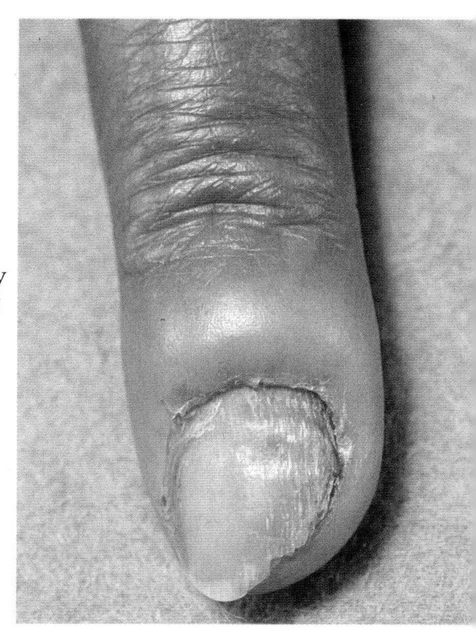

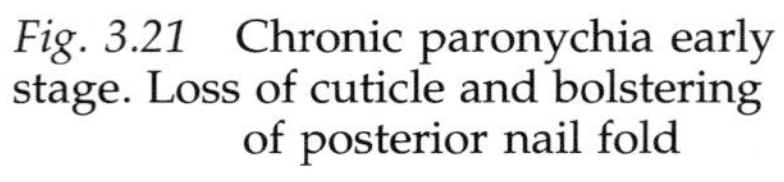

Fig. 3.21 Chronic paronychia early stage. Loss of cuticle and bolstering of posterior nail fold

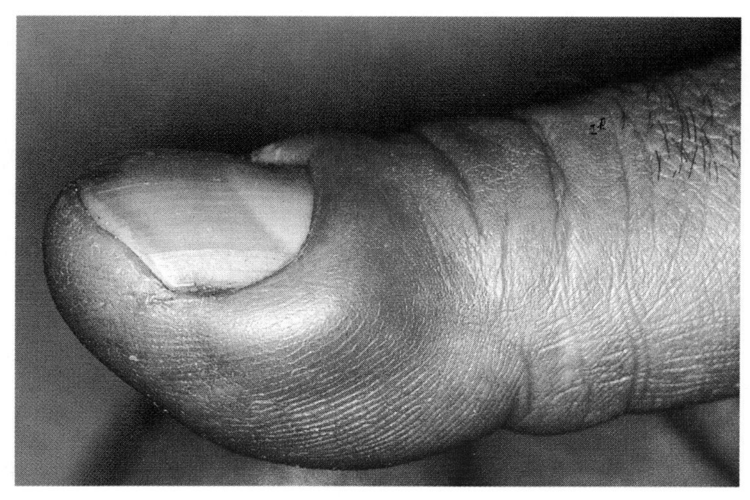

Fig. 3.22 Chronic paronychia. Note bolstering of nail folds

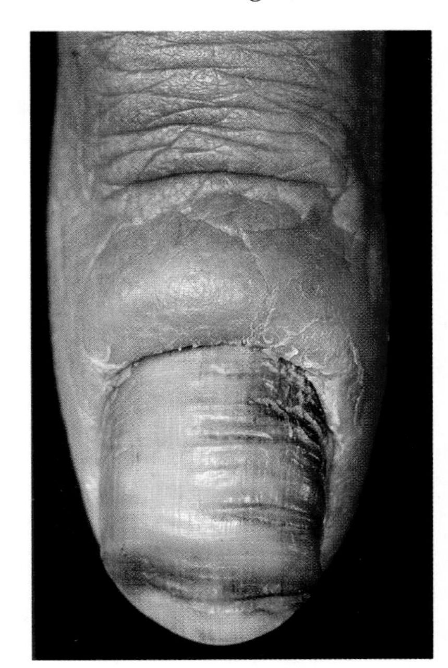

Fig. 3.23 Chronic paronychia producing cross ridging of nail plate

with allowing healing of the nail fold as well as removal of organisms. Some authors, such as Barlow *et al.* (1970) believe that the initial cause of nail fold damage is *S. aureus* in many cases. Stone and Mullins (1965) have shown that the process can also be initiated by introducing non-viable *C. albicans* into a non-infected nail fold. Hence it is possible that immunological damage may be involved in the process. In addition antigenic debris lodging within the enlarged nail fold space will act as a foreign body and lead to further chronic inflammation. In due course the nail fold becomes chronically thickened and bolstered with further loss of the cuticle.

In new cases of paronychia it is worth taking swabs from the nail fold and examining for yeasts by direct microscopy as well as culturing for both fungi and bacteria. Treatment consists of a number of ancillary measures in addition to specific therapy. These include:

(1) Patients should be advised to dry their hands carefully after wetting.

(2) They should not attempt to clean out their nail folds with sharpened sticks, as they may exacerbate the condition.

(3) They should wear gloves when doing the washing up.

(4) Skin disease affecting the nail folds such as eczema should be treated appropriately.

(5) The chronic infections should be treated by daily application of an imidazole or polyene antifungal lotion, such as econazole, or an antiseptic such as 4% thymol in chloroform or 15% sulphacetamide in 50% spirit (alcohol). There appears to be no particular advantage in using oral ketoconazole or itraconazole over topical agents as the latter are effective (Wong *et al.*, 1984). Treatment with antifungal/antiseptic agents has to be continued for several months until the nail fold has healed. Itraconazole is useful if there is secondary nail plate invasion by candida.

(6) In acute lesions or in exacerbations of chronic disease where *S. aureus* is isolated, oral therapy for 2 weeks with erythromycin or flucloxacillin is useful. Alternatively antibiotic sensitivity testing of bacteria isolated can be used to identify the appropriate therapy. If the lesion is pointing and pus is present it may need to be incised. However, there is no place for surgical removal of the nail under these circumstances. Gram-negative bacteria are best treated with antiseptic lotions, and topical aminoglycosides should be avoided. Successful treatment of chronic paronychia can occur without eradication of gram-negative bacteria (Wong *et al.*, 1984).

(7) Topical corticosteroid therapy may be helpful in chronic lesions, particularly if combined with an antifungal agent. However, creams or ointments should be carefully applied to the area as they may accumulate under the fold and contribute to the persistent inflammation. As a general principle the application of lotions is preferable.

References

Barlow, A J E, Chattaway, F W, Holgate, W C and Aldersley, T A (1970) Chronic paronychia. *Brit. J. Derm.* **82** 448

Belsan, I and Fragner, P (1965) Onychomykosen, lenorgerufen durch *Scopulariopsis brevicaulis. Der Hautartz* **16** 258

Davies, R R (1980) Griseofulvin. In: *Antifungal Chemotherapy*, ed. Speller, D C E. John Wiley and Sons, Chichester, p. 149

Davies, R R, Everall, J D and Hamilton, E (1967) Mycological and clinical evaluation of griseofulvin for chronic onychomycosis. *Brit. Med. J.* **3** 464
English, M (1976) Nails and fungi. *Brit. J. Derm.* **94** 697
Esteves, J (1959) Pathogenesis and treatment of chronic paronychia. *Dermatologica* **119** 229
Frain-Bell, W (1957) Chronic paronychia. Short review of 590 cases. *Trans. St John's Hosp. Derm. Soc.* **38** 29
Goodfield, M J D (1992) Short duration therapy with terbinafine for dermatophyte onychomycosis: a multi-centre study. *Brit. J. Derm.* **126 suppl 39** 33
Hay, R J and Clayton, Y M (1982) The treatment of patients with chronic mucocutaneous candidosis and candida onychomycosis with ketoconazole. *Clin. Exp. Derm.* **7** 155
Hay, R J and Moore, M K (1984) Clinical features of superficial fungal infections caused by *Hendersonula toruloidea* and *Scytalidium hyalinum. Brit. J. Derm.* **110** 677
Heiberg, J K and Svejgaard, E (1981) Toxic hepatitis during ketoconazole treatment. *Brit. Med. J.* **283** 825
Reinel, D (1992) Topical treatment of onychomycosis with amorolfine 5% nail lacquer: comparative efficacy and tolerability of once and twice weekly use. *Dermatology* **182 suppl** 21
Stone, O J and Mullins, J R (1965) Role of *Candida albicans* in chronic disease. *Arch. Derm.* **91** 70
Stone, O J and Mullins, F J (1968) Chronic paronychia in children. *Clin. Pediat.* **7** 104
Willemsen, M, de Doncker, P, Willems, J, *et al.* (1992) Post-treatment itraconazole levels in the nail; new implications for treatment. *J. Am. Acad. Derm.* **26** 731–735
Wong, E S M, Hay, R J, Clayton, Y M and Noble, W C (1984) Comparison of the therapeutic effect of ketoconazole tablets and econazole lotion in the treatment of chronic paronychia. *Clin. Exp. Derm.* **9** 489
Zaias, N (1966) Superficial white onychomycosis. *Sabouraudia* **5** 99
Zaias, N (1972) Onychomycosis. *Arch. Derm.* **105** 263

4

Psoriasis

P. D. Samman and D. A. Fenton

Psoriasis is one of the commonest skin diseases and the nails are involved in a high proportion of cases. In Crawford's series (Crawford, 1938) almost 50% of cases had nail involvement. If a single close inspection only is made about 25% of cases will show nail involvement but over a lifetime the incidence must be nearer 80–90%. Finger nails are said to be involved more often than toe nails (Zaias, 1969), but this may be apparent rather than real as toe nail involvement is seldom a cause for complaint. The nails may be involved in the complete absence of psoriasis elsewhere, and many of the worst cases of nail involvement show only minimal psoriasis in other areas. These minimal changes are most likely to be found in the scalp or on the genitalia. Psoriasis is thus the most important single cause of nail dystrophy.

Pitting

The nails are deformed in many ways. The feature most widely recognised is pitting. This may vary from a few isolated pits on one nail (Figs. 4.1, 4.2) to uniform pitting of all nails. The pits are usually small and seldom more than 1 mm across and quite shallow. Much larger pits and even punched-out areas are seen occasionally. The pits are generally found scattered irregularly over a few nails but occasionally are quite

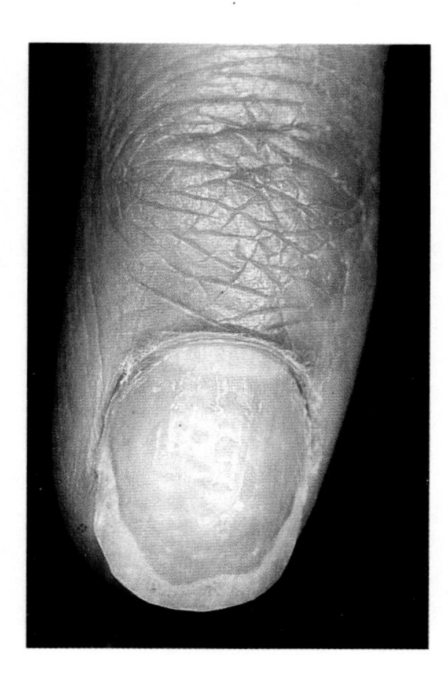

Fig. 4.1 Psoriasis—pitting

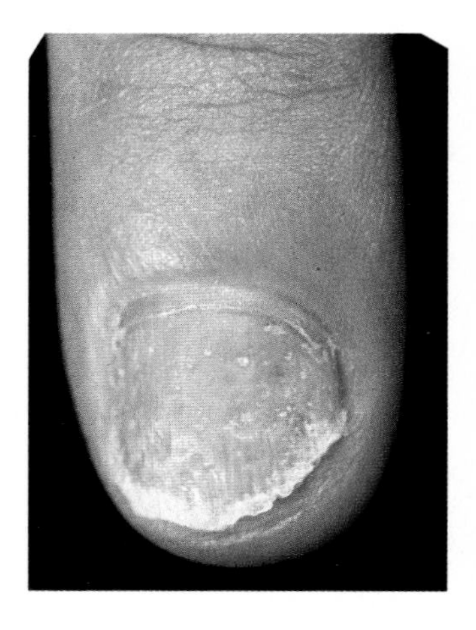

Fig. 4.2 Psoriasis—pitting

regular and form into lines of pits across the nails (Fig. 4.3). As they may also be produced at regular intervals the pits may form into lines in the long axis of the nails also. This type of regular pitting may also be seen occasionally in alopecia areata. Other common causes of irregular pitting of the nails are dermatitis and chronic paronychia but these conditions can usually be readily distinguished. Pits may, however, appear without evidence of skin disease, but are normally very insignificant in such cases. Mottling in the half moon (lunula) is often seen in association with pitting in psoriasis

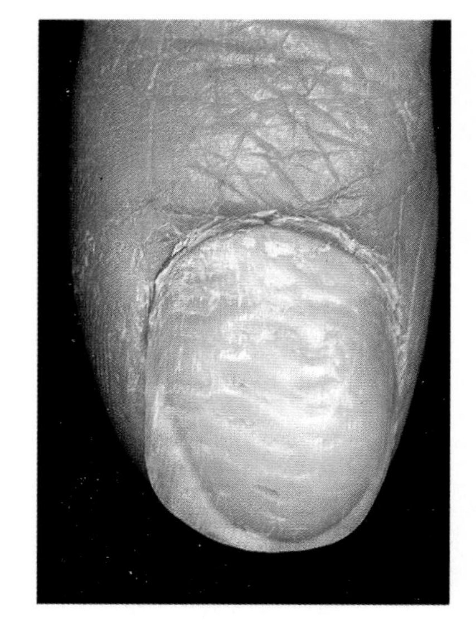

Fig. 4.3 Psoriasis—transverse ridging and rippling

and sometimes with pitting from other causes, such as alopecia areata.

Alkiewiez (1948) showed that the pits are due to retention of nuclei (parakeratosis) in parts of the nail keratin. These areas are weaker than the surrounding normal keratin and may be shed leaving the pits on the nail surface. Zaias (1969) has shown more exactly how this occurs. A scanning electron microscopic study of normal and psoriatic nails (Mauro, Lumpkin and Danzig, 1975) has shown that the surface of normal nails is made up of overlapping flat cells with the overlap opposite to the direction of growth. The cell surfaces are generally flat and closely opposed. A few micropits are visible. The pits of psoriatic nails differ from normal nails in that the cells on the surface are smaller and do not have the overlapping pattern. They appear to be heaped up, to be growing in a haphazard way and to be crowded together, with spaces between the poorly interdigitated cells. Numerous micropits are also seen.

Onycholysis

Onycholysis, or separation of the nail from its bed is not so well recognised as part of psoriasis but occurs almost as often as pitting. The separation is usually partial and involves one or several nails. It most commonly starts at the free edge of the nail but may commence in the centre of the nail plate. Onycholysis occurs in many conditions other than psoriasis but in the latter there is usually a yellow margin visible between the pink normal nail and the white separated area. If the separation starts in the middle of the nail the yellow margin will form into a complete ring. Smaller yellow patches are sometimes called salmon patches or oil drops (Figs. 4.4, 4.5). Although not pathognomonic of psoriasis this yellow colour is only seen occasionally in lysis from other causes. Onycholysis may come on quite suddenly in psoriasis and many nails may become involved overnight. It is apparent therefore that it is due to an alteration in the nail bed and not to changes occurring in the matrix area. Subungual hyperkeratosis is often present (Fig. 4.6).

A further change seen occasionally is apparently a complication of severe onycholysis. The proximal part of the nail bed with the nail still attached becomes raised above the distal part so that the nail is very widely separated and, for comfort, the patient is then forced to cut the nail very

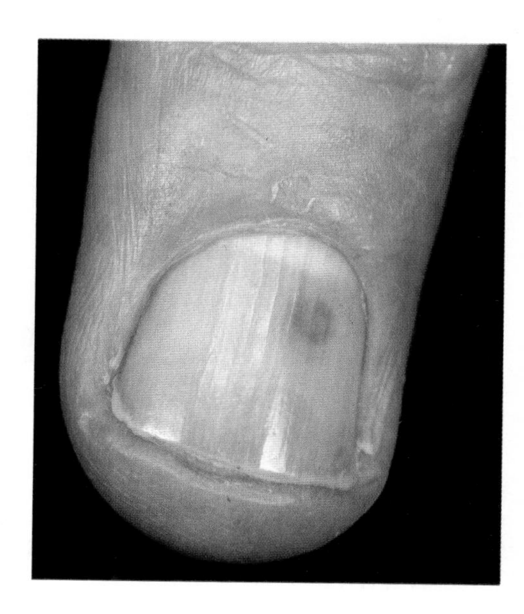

Fig. 4.4 Psoriasis—'oil drop' onycholysis

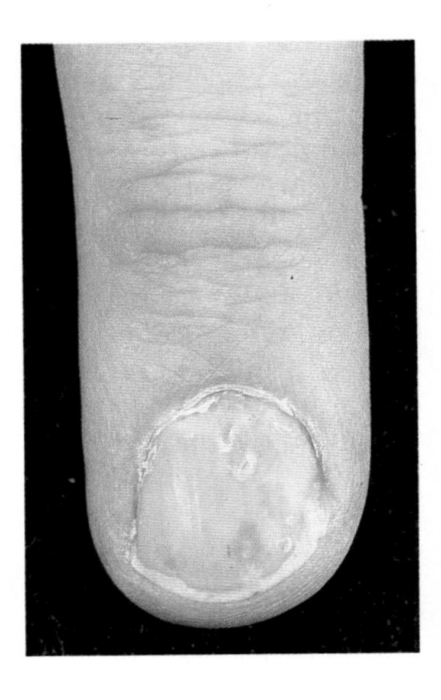

Fig. 4.5 Psoriasis—pits and 'salmon patches'

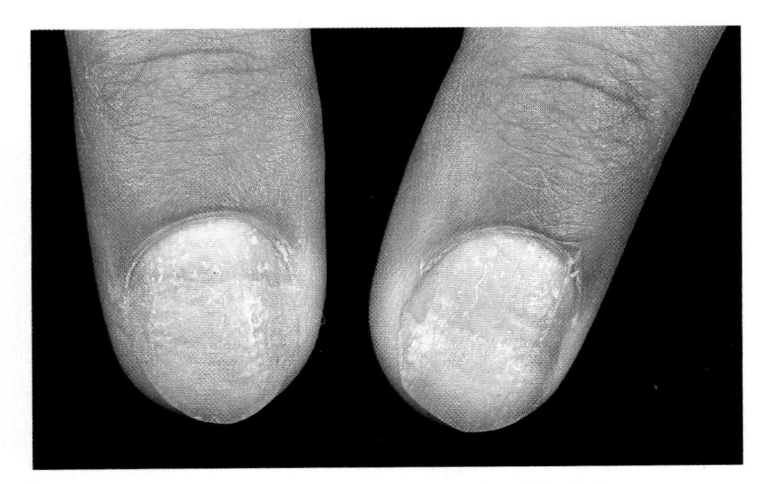

Fig. 4.6 Onycholysis in psoriasis with pitting

short (Fig. 4.7). Psoriasis is probably the most common cause of onycholysis, but it may occur under many other circumstances (pp. 25 and 116). Roughening of the nail plate surface (trachyonychia) (Fig. 4.8) and splinter haemorrhages (Fig. 4.9) are often seen.

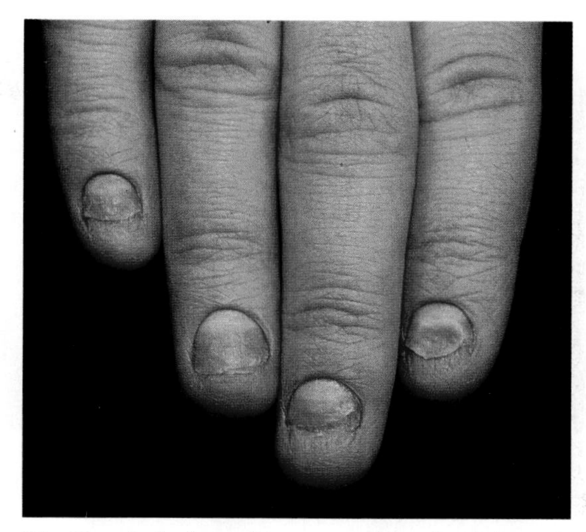

Fig. 4.7 Onycholysis—wide separation of nail from its bed

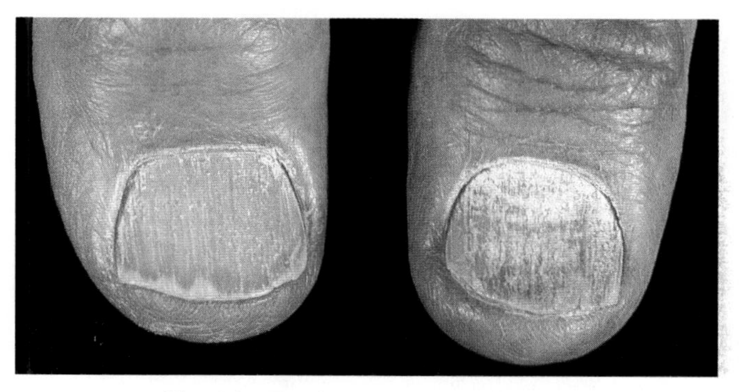

Fig. 4.8 Trachyonychia in psoriasis

Abnormality of the nail plate

The third and most distressing change in the nails seen in psoriasis is a grosser abnormality of the nail plate. The nail loses its lustre, becomes opaque, discoloured, irregular and may be thickened. The process may be seen to start as the nail emerges from under the cuticle and moves forward as the nail grows to involve the whole nail plate (Fig. 4.10). One or several nails may be involved and not necessarily all

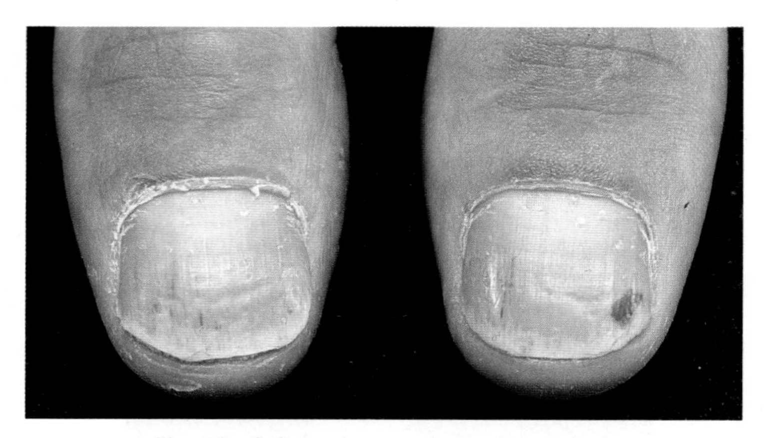

Fig. 4.9 Splinter haemorrhages in psoriasis

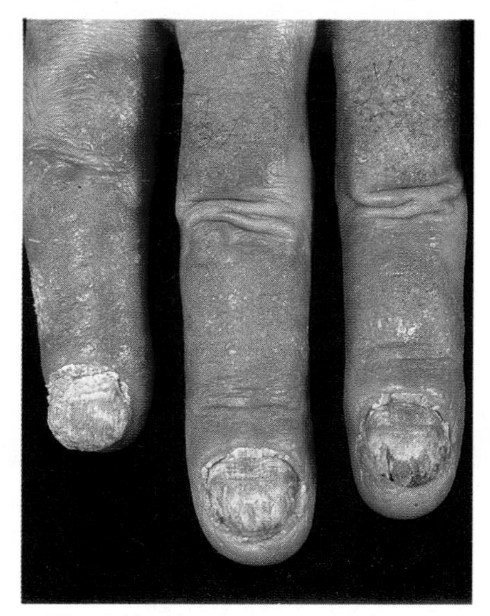

Fig. 4.10 Psoriasis—gross changes

to the same extent. Often, however, by the time the patient reports most nails are totally involved. It is apparent that this type of change is dependent on abnormalities in the matrix area. The deformity is not static but may show constant change, one nail returning to normal whilst others become involved. This changing pattern is seldom seen with other nail disorders. Zaias (1969) says that the colour change is due to large amounts of a serum-like exudate containing glycoprotein which accumulates in and under the affected nails; the glycoprotein is commonly found in inflammatory and eczematous diseases affecting the nail bed but not in fungal infections. Part of the colour change is, however, due to minute haemorrhages in the nail bed visible through the nail plate.

Fungal infection

The only important differential diagnosis in this third type of deformity is fungal or candidial infection of the nail plate. The colour and irregularity may be seen in either, and subungual haemorrhages may occur in either. With fungal infections however it is always possible to find the organism in potash preparations and the nail plate is usually softer than in psoriasis. Leyden *et al.* (1972) describe a method of examining nail shavings and subungual hyperkeratosis to show up parakeratotic cells in psoriasis which they did not find in other nail disorders except for occasional nucleated cells in onychomycosis.

Dermatophytes

Very seldom are dermatophytes found in association with nail psoriasis although yeasts and bacteria are commonly present in the subungual debris (Zaias, 1969), and it has been pointed out that chronic paronychia (Chapter 3) is commonly found in association with nail psoriasis (Ganor, 1975).

Other deformities

Great thickening of the nail is another less common change in psoriasis. The appearances are similar to those just described except that the nail is greatly thickened by incorporation of much material from the nail bed into the nail (ventral nail). This is more often found in toe nails than in finger nails. A similar change is found occasionally in Darier's disease and in pachyonychia congenita.

The formation of hard material at the edge of the nail lifting the nail from its bed and distorting the nail plate is another feature of psoriasis which may occur in association with, or independently of the other conditions described. Overcurvature of one or more nails may be seen occasionally (Fig. 4.11).

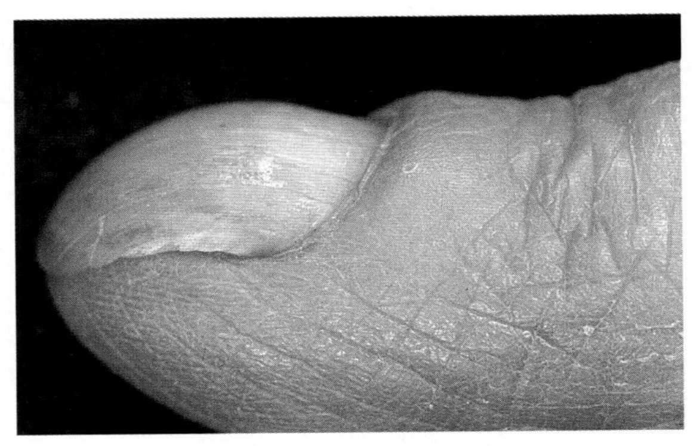

Fig. 4.11 Psoriasis—overcurvature of the nail

Histological changes

Lewin, DeWit and Ferrington (1972) investigated the histological changes in the nail matrix and nail bed in psoriasis and showed that there was a metaplastic change in both areas producing a skin-like epithelium so that the histology resembled that of normal skin.

Arthropathy

Arthropathy involving the distal interphalangeal joints may occur with severe nail psoriasis (Figs. 4.12, 4.13), but is rare compared with the number of cases where the nails are involved without arthritis. The arthritis is of a destructive type but is almost certainly not the same as rheumatoid arthritis. X-ray will show the joint changes and there is often destruction of the distal phalanx. The Rose-Waaler test is negative.

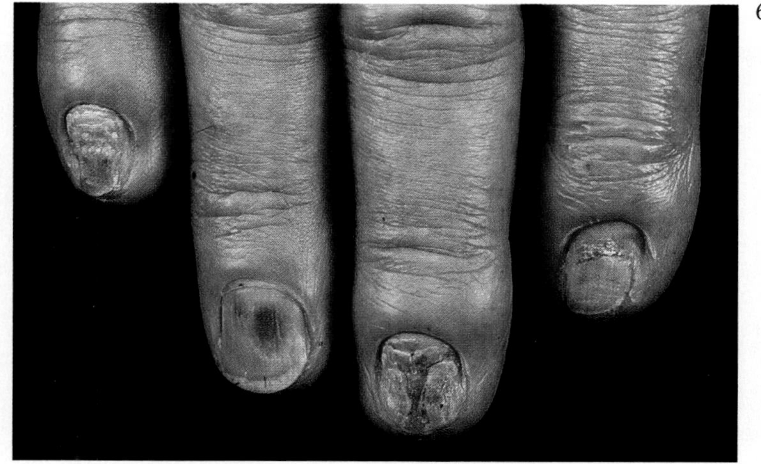

Fig. 4.12(a) Psoriasis of nails and arthropathy of distal interphalangeal joints

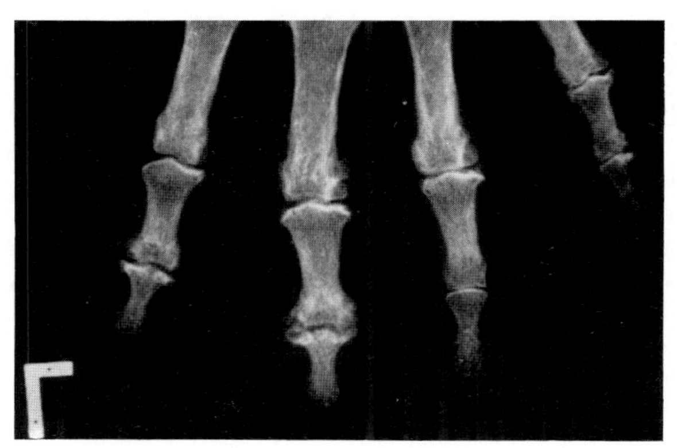

Fig. 4.12(b) Radiograph showing arthropathy of distal interphalangeal joints

Treatment

Treatment of psoriasis of the nails is unsatisfactory. The condition often improves spontaneously and may improve as skin lesions resolve with or without treatment. Improvement of the severe type of change will usually occur following injections of triamcinolone into the matrix area but the improvement is normally short lived unless the injections are repeated. Needle injections are, however, painful but the use of the 'Porton gun' (Abell, 1972) or similar apparatus is not recom-

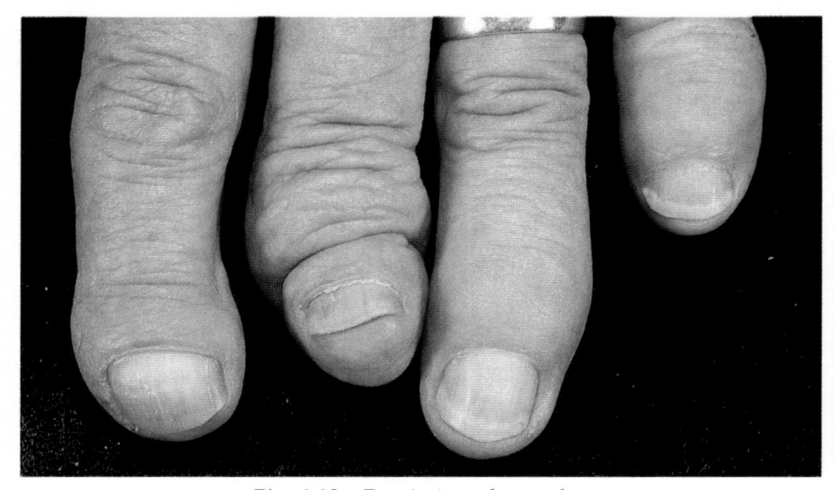

Fig. 4.13 Psoriatic arthropathy

mended owing to the difficulty in sterilising the apparatus; it is theoretically possible to transfer a viral infection from one patient to the next with the gun. Intralesional steroid injections can occasionally cause subungual haematoma (Scher, 1985). The application of 0.025% fluocinolone acetonide cream or other fluorinated topical steroid creams under polythene occlusion is worthy of trial. It produces improvement in some cases where the nails are badly affected but must not be repeated indefinitely or atrophy of the soft tissues around the nail will occur. Fredericsson (1974) obtained useful improvement from the topical application of 1% fluorouracil solution without occlusion over a period of 6 months; about 25 ml of the solution was used each month. Pitting and subungual hyperkeratosis respond better than onycholysis (which may worsen). Abraham and Fluerman (1978) used a 2% solution. X-ray therapy will occasionally induce a remission which may last months or years and may therefore be tried if other methods fail. The dose required is 1 Gy at 60 or 70 kV repeated at weekly intervals to a total of 4 or 5 Gy. The nail beds do not stand a great deal of X-ray therapy so the treatment should not be repeated more than once or twice in the patient's lifetime. Onycholysis is seldom improved by this treatment. In the great majority of cases the best treatment is to reassure the patient in the hope that a spontaneous remission may occur.

Local PUVA cleared pitting and onycholysis in two out of five patients using a 1% 8-methoxypsoralen application, but relapse occurred 4 to 8 months later (Handfield-Jones, Boyle and Harman, 1987). Oral photochemotherapy (Marx and Scher, 1980) can also help; subungual photohaemolysis is an occasional application. Systemic retinoids, including both etretinate and acitretin, are sometimes helpful (Rabinowitz, Scher and Shupack, 1983) although again relapse occurs on discontinuing therapy.

Pustular psoriasis and acrodermatitis continua

The nail changes in these conditions are the same as the grosser changes in psoriasis and it is probable that they are all variants of the same process (Figs. 4.14, 4.15). Pustules forming under a nail may occasionally result in permanent loss of the nail.

The author has published details of a case of generalised pustular psoriasis (Samman, 1961) in whom all the finger nails were grossly distorted and thickened (Fig. 4.16). When given treatment with systemic triamcinolone the portion of nail derived from the matrix was shed from each finger and

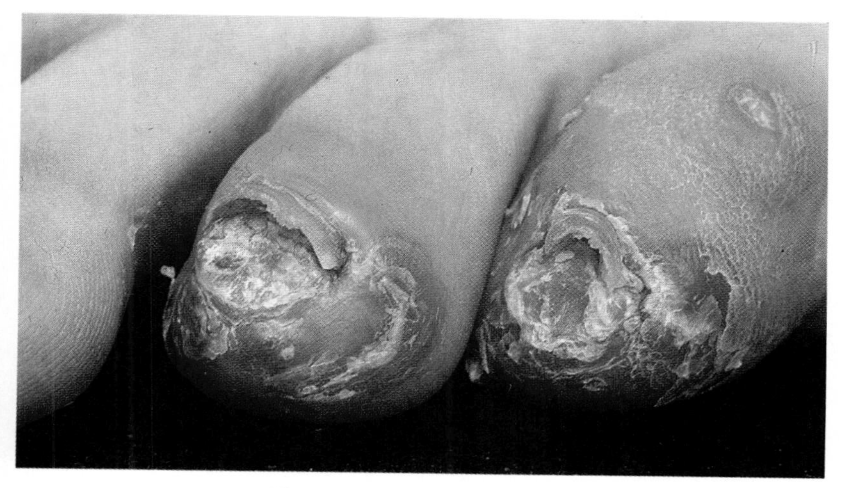

Fig. 4.14 Pustular psoriasis

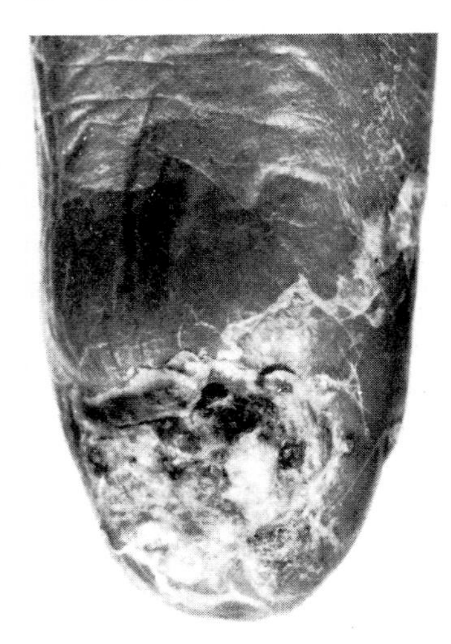

Fig. 4.15 Acrodermatitis

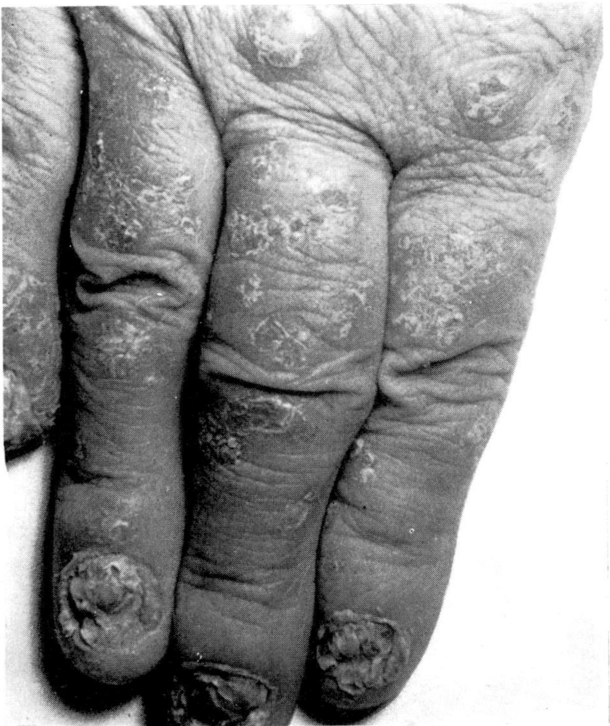

Fig. 4.16 Pustular psoriasis before shedding main part of nails

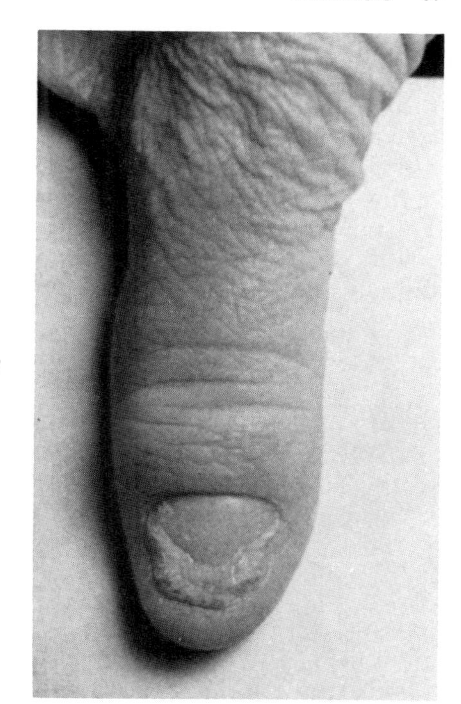

Fig. 4.17 Pustular psoriasis after shedding main part of nails

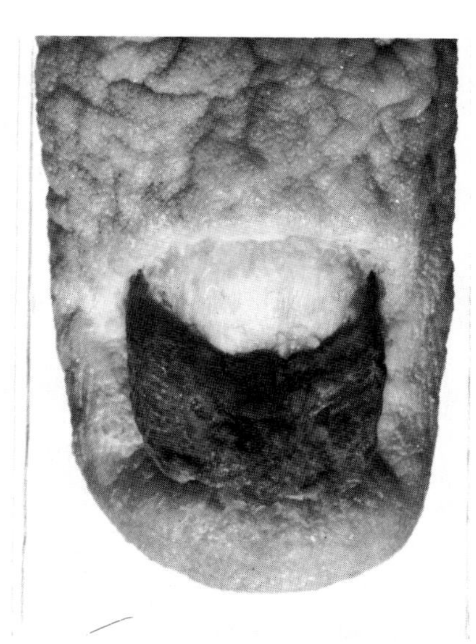

Fig. 4.18 Same patient as *Figs. 4.16, 4.17*—post mortem

was not replaced, so that the nail folds remained empty. Hard keratin arising from the nail bed however remained *in situ* and formed a satisfactory nail (Figs. 4.17, 4.18). The portion remaining corresponded to Lewis's ventral nail and appeared quite different from the pseudo-nail which may cover the nail bed if a nail is surgically removed and the matrix destroyed. The ventral nail here was presumably a development from the sole horn (p. 5). The histological appearances of one of these digits is shown in Figs. 4.19 and 4.20.

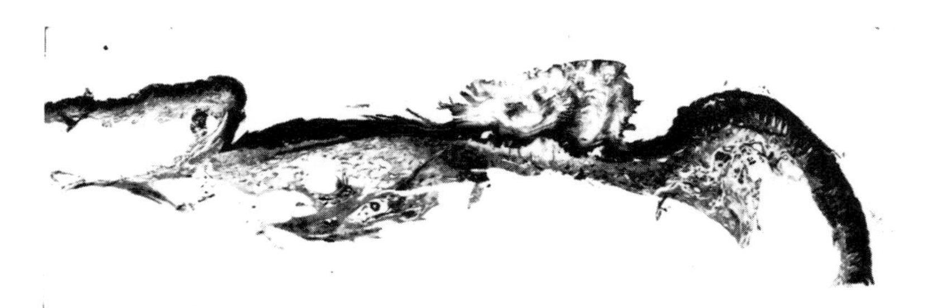

Fig. 4.19 Low power photomicrograph (×5) anteroposterior through nail shown in *Fig. 4.18*

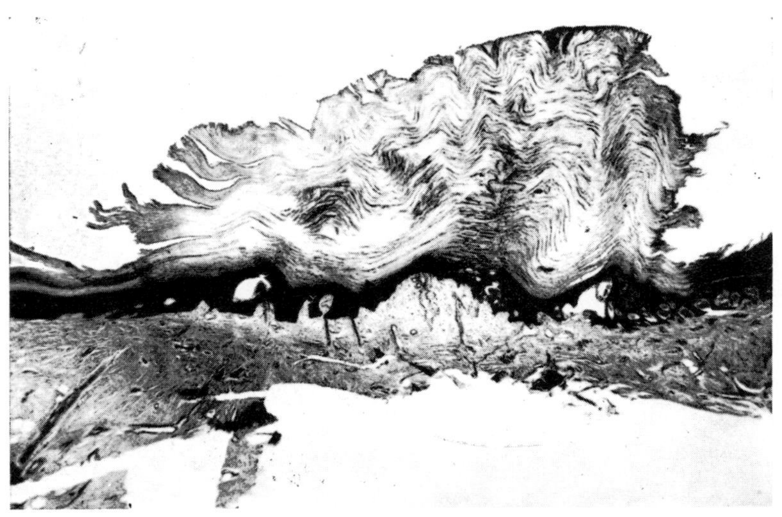

Fig. 4.20 High power photomicrograph (×17) showing details of 'ventral nail' or 'sole horn'

References

Abell, E (1972) Treatment of psoriatic nail dystrophy. *Brit. J. Derm.* **86** 79
Abraham, D and Fluerman, E J (1978) Local treatment of psoriatic nails with 5 fluorouracil 2% solution. *Harefuah* **94** 367
Alkiewicz, J (1948) Psoriasis of the nail. *Brit. J. Derm.* **60** 196
Crawford, G M (1938) Psoriasis of the nails. *Arch. Derm. Syph.* **38** 583
Fredericsson, G M (1938) Psoriasis of the nails. *Arch. Derm. Syph.* **38** 583
Fredericsson, T (1974) Topically applied fluorouracil in treatment of psoriatic nails. *Arch. Derm.* **110** 735
Ganor, S (1975) Chronic paronychia and psoriasis. *Brit. J. Derm.* **92** 685
Handfield-Jones, S E, Boyle, J and Harman R R M (1987) Local PUVA treatment for nail psoriasis. *Brit. J. Derm.* **116** 280
Lewin, K, DeWit, S and Ferrington, R A (1972) Pathology of the finger nail in psoriasis. *Brit. J. Derm.* **86** 555
Leyden, J L, Dechard, J W and Goldschmidt, H (1972) Exfoliative cytology in the diagnosis of psoriasis of the nails. *Cutis* **10** 701
Marx, J L, Scher, R K (1980) Response of psoriatic nails to oral photochemotherapy. *Arch. Derm.* **116** 1023
Mauro, J, Lumpkin, L R and Danzig, P I (1975) Scanning electron microscopy of psoriatic nail pits. *NY State J. Med.* **75** 339
Rabinowitz, A S, Scher, R K and Shupack, J T (1983) Response of psoriatic nails to aromatic retinoid etretinate. *Arch. Derm.* **119** 627
Samman, P D (1961) The ventral nail. *Arch. Derm. Syph.* **84** 1030
Scher, R K (1985) Psoriasis of the nail. *Derm. Clin.* **3** 387
Zaias, N (1969) Psoriasis of the nail. *Arch. Derm.* **99** 567

5

Nail disorders associated with other dermatological conditions

P. D. Samman and D. A. Fenton

Dermatitis

Dermatitis can play havoc with the nails and in most cases the cause of the nail damage is obvious. At times, however, the dermatitis is under control before the patient complains of the nail changes and in these one has to rely on the history for confirmatory diagnosis. Such patients are usually referred as having suspected fungal infection of the nails; this is generally easily excluded.

Nail changes may occur in any type of dermatitis involving the hands and in particular the skin adjacent to the nail, but atopic dermatitis more frequently affects the nails than do other types. In atopic dermatitis and in pompholyx the nail changes sometimes predominate. One must assume in these cases that the eczematous process is most marked on the under-surface of the dorsal nail fold.

The usual change is an atrophic process and consists of the development of irregular ridges across the nail (Figs. 5.1, 5.2). In addition coarse pitting may affect one or more nails. The ridges occur independently on one or several nails and the overall change is a very ugly nail. If the ridges go deep enough they may lead to temporary shedding of part of

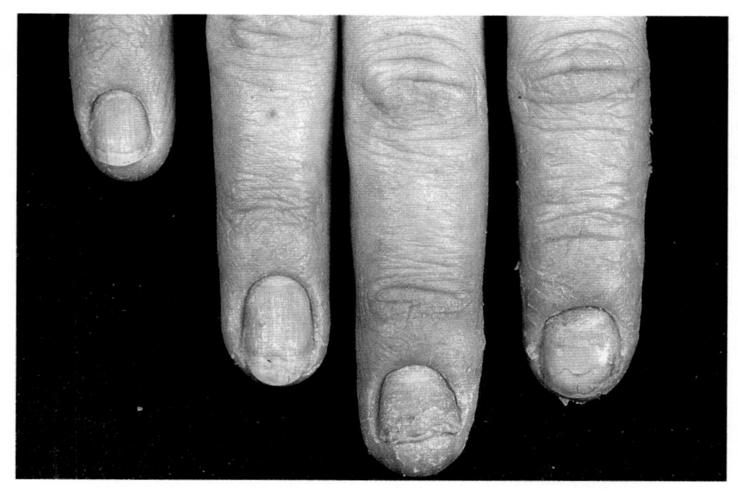

Fig. 5.1 Atopic eczema—course pitting and cross ridging

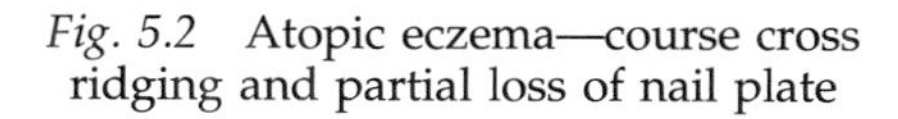

Fig. 5.2 Atopic eczema—course cross ridging and partial loss of nail plate

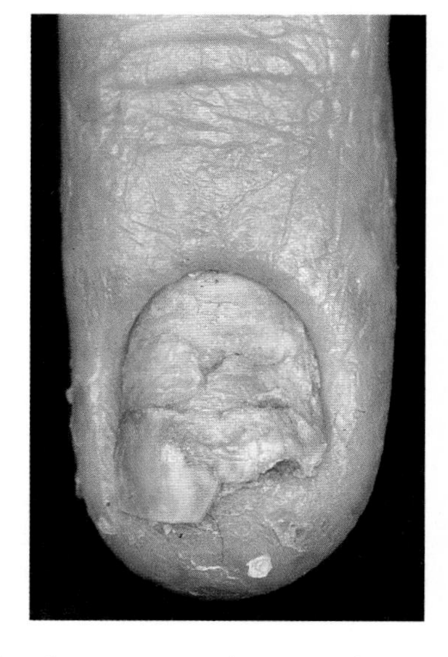

the nail. In the early stages only the proximal part of the nails will be involved. Subungual haemorrhages, either petechial or more extensive, may complicate the picture, as may chronic paronychia. The ridges must be distinguished from ridges formed by other causes and in particular the traumatic nail dystrophy produced by a habit tic (p. 155).

The sudden onset of generalised dermatitis may be accompanied by the formation of a depression on all nails similar to Beau's lines (p. 115), but in dermatitis the nail behind the depression is likely to be deformed (Fig. 5.3). In exfoliative dermatitis the nails may be shed.

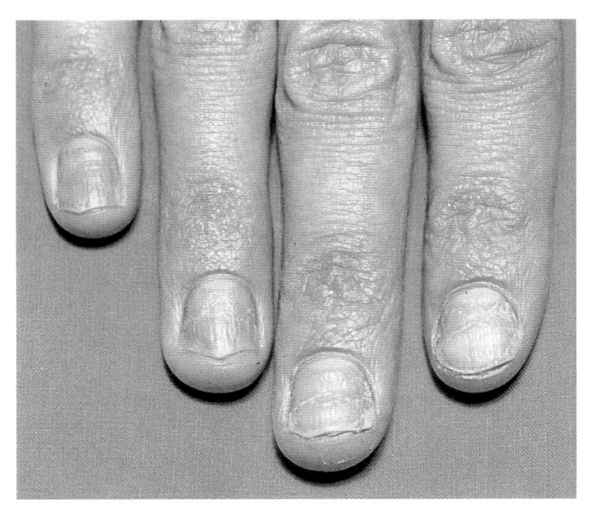

Fig. 5.3 The nails following the onset of generalised dermatitis—depression on all nails followed by deformed nails

Although the usual nail change in dermatitis is an atrophic process (Fig. 5.4), occasionally gross hypertrophy occurs. These cases are associated with inflammation of the nail fold, and the nail becomes very thick and irregular (Figs. 5.5, 5.6). This type of hypertrophy is probably always due to exogenous causes. It must be distinguished from psoriasis precipitated by trauma or chemical irritation. In these cases there will be no evidence of dermatitis of the fingers but there may also be no other evidence of psoriasis. Dermatitis of the nails is often mistaken for onychomycosis but it can readily be differentiated by the absence of fungal mycelia in nail clippings. When fungi are present onychomycosis can be diagnosed with certainty and the result of treatment with griseofulvin

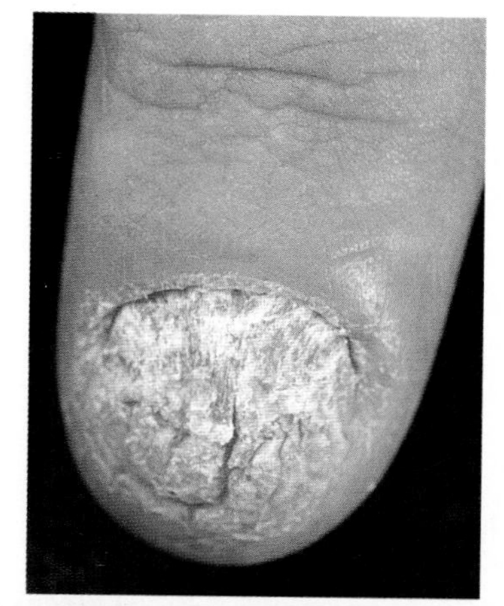

Fig. 5.4 Nail destruction in contact dermatitis

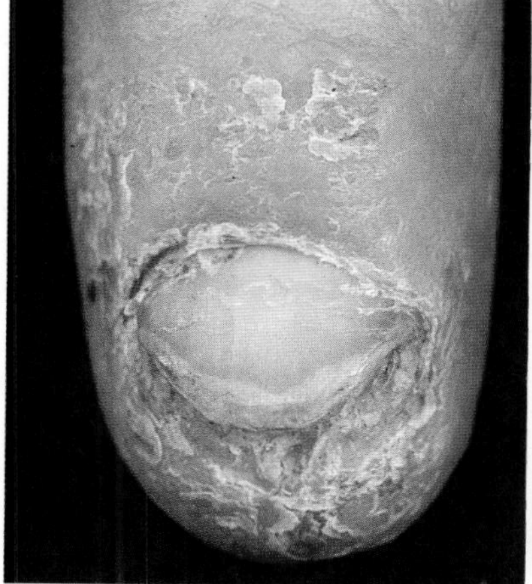

Fig. 5.5 Contact dermatitis

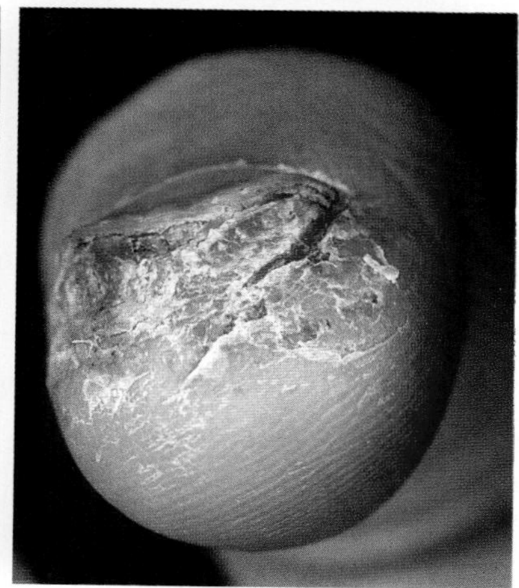

Fig. 5.6 Contact dermatitis—nail hypertrophy

or terbinafine confirms this finding. Psoriasis can usually be differentiated on clinical grounds.

Onycholysis is not infrequently seen in association with dermatitis of the fingertips, presumably as a result of irritant material being trapped under the free edge of the nail and then penetrating further distally. Occasionally the irritant material may pass through the nail plate to reach the nail bed. Shelley (1972) has noted onycholysis from the topical application of 5% 5-fluorouracil to the fingertips under occlusion. The condition was reversible and was not produced by a 2% preparation.

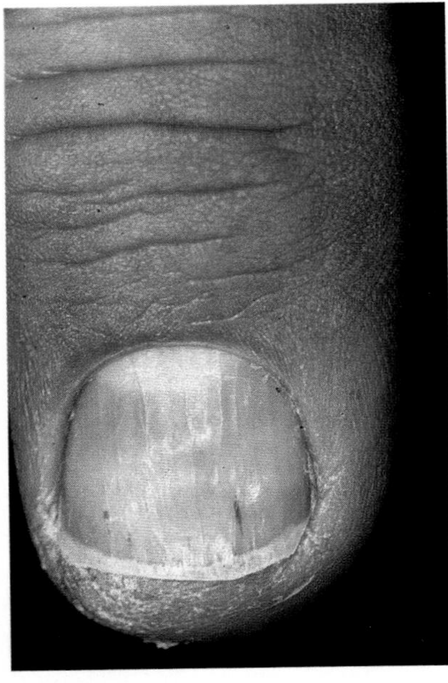

Fig. 5.7 Splinter haemorrhages in dermatitis

Koilonychia may be associated with use of organic solvents and motor oils (Fisher, 1986).

Both irritant and allergic contact reactions may result from use of nail cosmetics, providing a variety of nail abnormalities (see Chapter 9).

Highly polished nails are sometimes seen in patients with generalised eczema (Fig. 5.7) or erythroderma. This is, of course, an indirect effect as the patients rub their hands on their skin to obtain relief from itching, preferring this to actual scratching as it does less damage. Another change sometimes encountered is the so called 'usure des ongles', a wearing away of the nails due to scratching.

Treatment is essentially treatment of the dermatitis. The nails will return to normal gradually, but complete restoration cannot be expected in less than 3 months. If chronic paronychia complicates the dermatitis it must be treated independently.

Lichen striatus

This is essentially an eczematous process in which the changes are restricted to a linear band often transversing

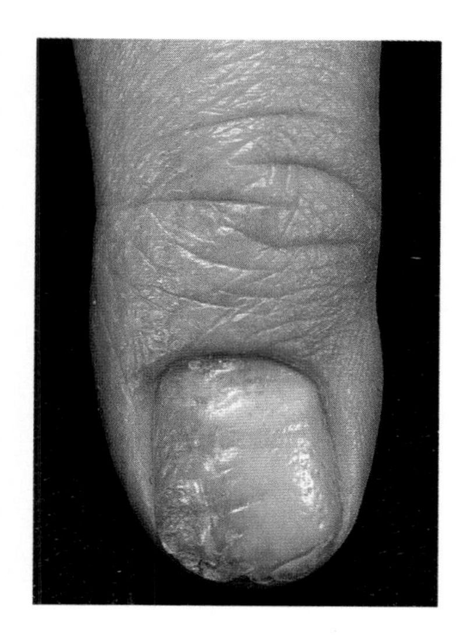

Fig. 5.8 Nail plate changes in lichen striatus

the whole length of a limb. If it extends as far as the distal phalanx it may cause changes in the nail of the affected digit similar to the changes seen in dermatitis (Fig. 5.8). These include hyperpigmentation (Zaias, 1980), leukonychia, onycholysis, shedding and splitting. Occasionally nail plate abnormality may persist for several years (Niren, Waldman and Barsky, 1981). It is usually restricted to a single finger. The author has seen a number of these cases but there are very few recorded in the literature. Baran *et al.* (1979) have collected four cases from the literature and describe four of their own. Kaufman (1974) describes one case.

Lichen planus

Samman (1961) has shown that some nail changes occur in about 10% of cases of lichen planus but that the damage is usually mild and transient. Permanent loss with scarring may, however, occur in a small percentage of cases. The commonest change seen on the nails in lichen planus is an increase in the longitudinal striations of the nail plate. The ridges may be accompanied by slight depressions on the surface which catch the light (Fig. 5.9). Ridging usually occurs in severe generalised lichen planus and may be seen starting near the cuticle and moving forward with the growth of the nail. The nail plate is often slightly thinned but after a time returns to normal. If the nail thinning is more severe the cuticle may grow forward over the base of the nail and attach itself to the nail plate (Fig. 5.10). An exaggeration of this process leads to pterygium formation (Figs. 5.11, 5.12) and may progress to permanent loss of the whole or a part of the nail. Permanent loss, however, is not necessarily preceded by pterygium formation. Temporary shedding of one or more nails is also encountered at times and the new nail when it forms may be incomplete. Nail loss can occur on any nail but most often it is the great toe nail.

Lichen planus of the nails without evidence of lichen planus elsewhere undoubtedly occurs (Burgoon and Kostrazewa, 1969; Cornelius and Shelley, 1967) and has been seen by the author on a number of occasions. Lichen planus in childhood is uncommon but several examples of nail destruction in children due to lichen planus have been seen by the author (Marks and Samman, 1972). The excess ridging of lichen planus can at times be mistaken for the 20-nail dystrophy (Scher, Fischbein and Ackerman, 1978). There is a rare variety of lichen planus which produces an atrophic process on the sole and permanent destruction of many toe nails (Figs. 5.13, 5.14).

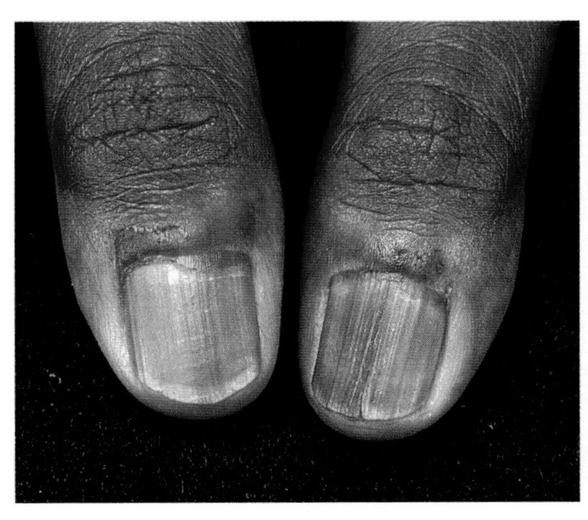

Fig. 5.9 Lichen planus—longitudinal ridging and depressions on nail surface with hyperpigmentation of nail bed

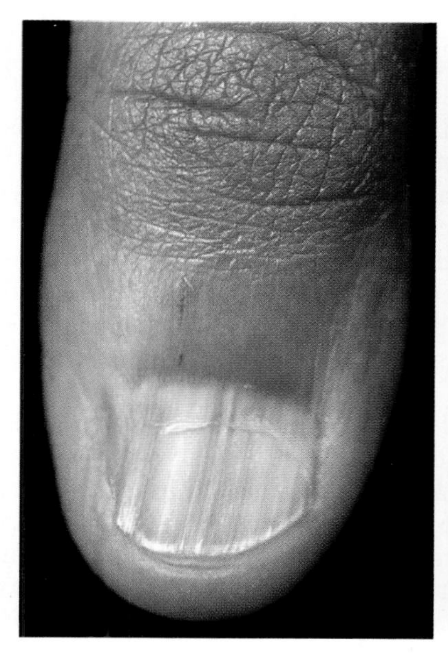

Fig. 5.10 Lichen planus—variable thinning, increased longitudinal striations of nail plate and forward growth of cuticle

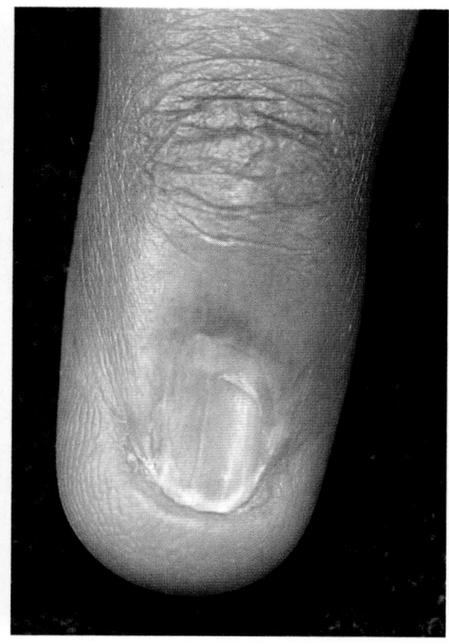

Fig. 5.11 Lichen planus—pterygium formation

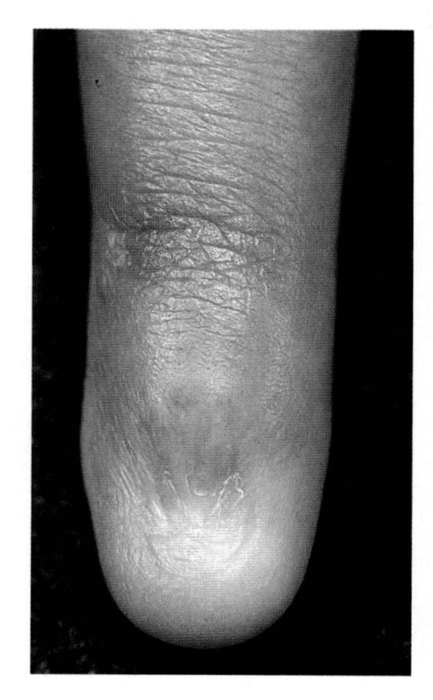

Fig. 5.12 Lichen planus—pterygium and nail atrophy

There may be very little evidence of lichen planus on other parts of the body (Cram, Kierland and Winkelmann, 1966; Degos and Schnitzler, 1967).

It can be shown histologically that the damage to the nail is the result of lichen planus in the region of the matrix and when scarring occurs it is analogous to the scarring seen following lichen planus around the hair roots. Zaias (1970) has shown that pterygium formation is due to an adhesion forming between the epidermis of the dorsal nail fold and the nail bed. He also says that lichen planus of the nail bed may give rise to hyperpigmentation, subungual hyperkeratosis and onycholysis.

Treatment for mild cases of nail change is unnecessary. For more severe cases local potent fluorinated topical steroid preparations may be helpful. Intralesional steroids may, however, also be required. If it is possible to make a diagnosis of lichen planus while severe nail changes are taking place, treatment with systemic corticosteroids may be justified in an attempt to save the nails. The possible harmful effects must be balanced against the chance of saving the nails, and in this context it should be realised that permanent damage to the nails can occur quite quickly. Prednisone, prednisolone or similar preparations may be used and the dose recommended is 15–20 mg daily for about 6 weeks and then gradual reduction

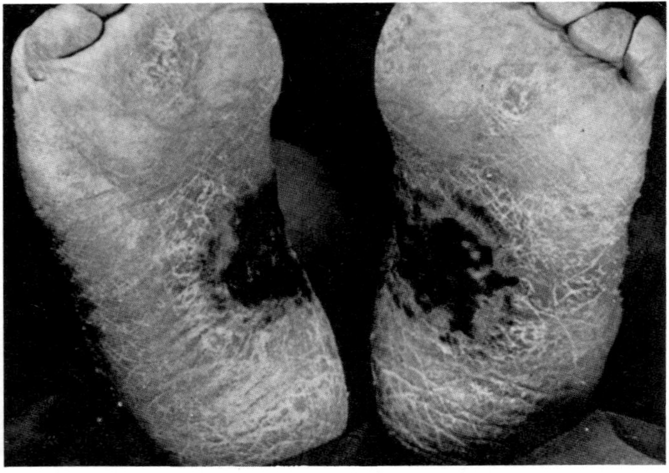

Fig. 5.13 Lichen planus—atrophic type affecting soles of feet

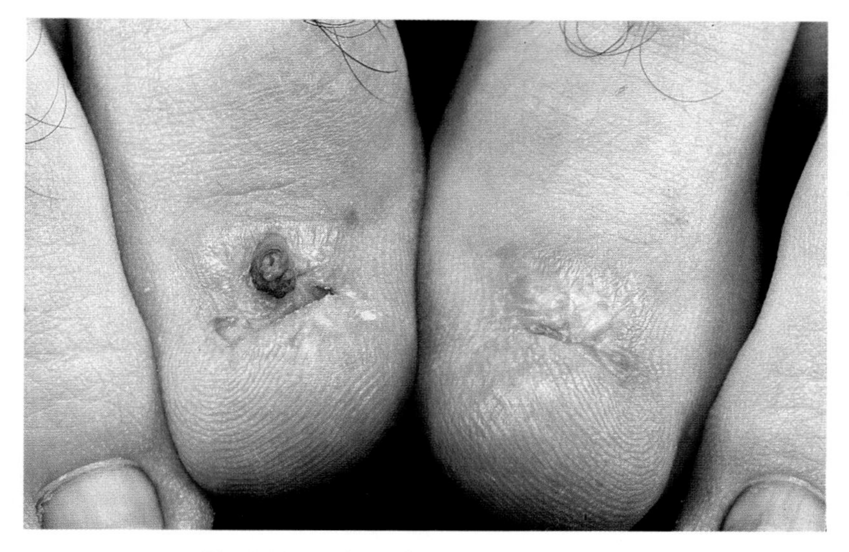

Fig. 5.14 Lichen planus—nail destruction

until the drug can be withdrawn after 3 months. The dose for children should be adjusted according to size of child.

Darier's disease

In this rare genetically determined disorder the nails are affected in a high percentage of cases. There have been a number of good descriptive papers (Ronchese, 1965; Schubert, 1966; Savin and Samman, 1970) on this disease. The nails may show a variety of changes, the most characteristic being the presence of a white streak or streaks (Fig. 5.15) extending longitudinally through the nail and crossing the half moon. One or more nails may be affected. Later the streaks lose their white colour and become darker and ridges may appear on the nails which then tend to crack (Fig. 5.16). Where a streak meets the free edge of the nail a V-shaped notch may appear (Fig. 5.17), and much less often the nail becomes greatly thickened (Fig. 5.18). Ronchese (1965) suggests that at times nail changes may occur in the absence of other evidence of the disease. This is one of the few occasions when a biopsy may be helpful in diagnosis as characteristic changes may be found in the nail folds and nail matrix (Zaias and Ackerman, 1973).

Treatment of the nail changes in Darier's disease is unsatisfactory; although the cutaneous lesions may improve with etretinate, nails usually do not (Burge *et al.*, 1981).

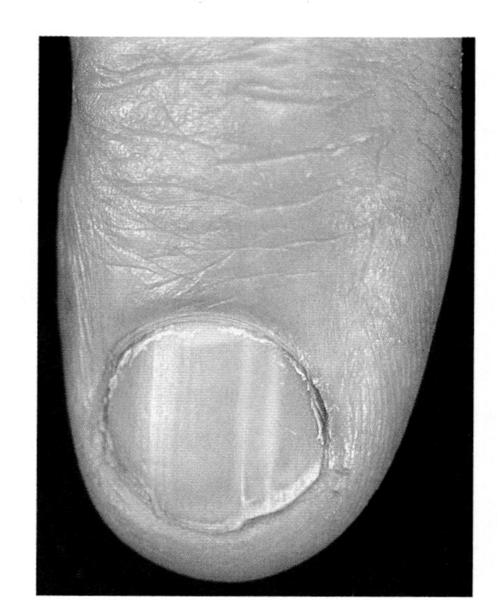

Fig. 5.15 Darier's disease—Characteristic white streaks

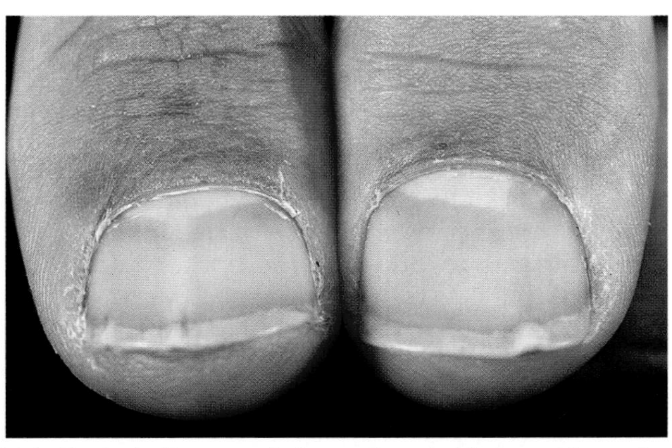

Fig. 5.16 Darier's disease—dark streak and ridging with notch at free margin

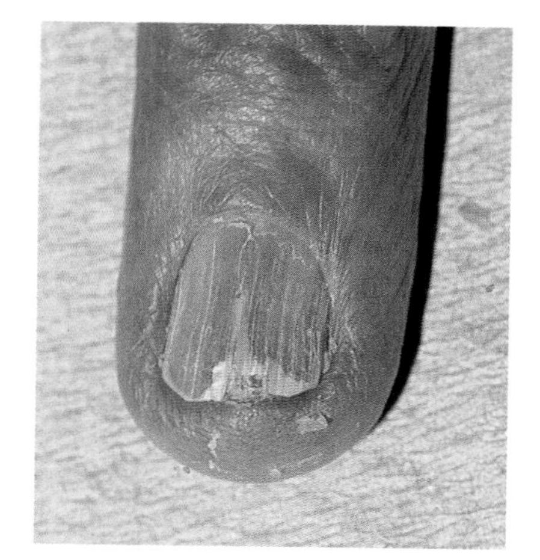

Fig. 5.17 Darier's disease—'V' - shaped notch at free edge and cracking

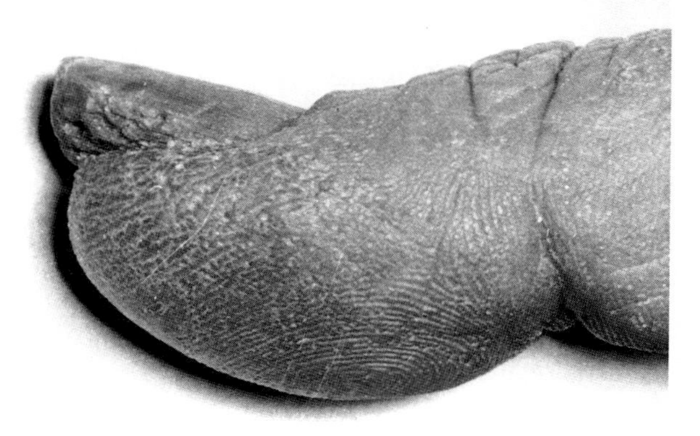

Fig. 5.18 Darier's disease—gross thickening

Alopecia areata

Shedding of the nails in alopecia areata is very uncommon. Some alteration of the nail plate is, however, quite frequent and in cases observed by one of us about 10% have shown some change. Rubisz Brzerzinska and Seferowicz (1974) say they found pits in 62% of 100 patients and other trophic changes in 4%. The common abnormality is pitting and the most characteristic is a uniform pitting affecting several nails (Figs. 5.19, 5.20). The pits are small as in psoriasis, but superficial, and when uniform make lines of pits both across and in the long axis of the nail. If the pits are produced very rapidly greater distortion of the nail plate occurs, the nail loses its lustre and becomes roughened (trachyonychia) (Fig. 5.21). Ganor (1977) suggests that psoriasis and alopecia areata occur together in many cases and that the pitting is really due to overt or hidden psoriasis. In nails with an exposed half moon there may be a meshwork of a pale yellow and pink colour visible through the nail plate in this area (Fig. 5.22) as seen also in psoriasis. Shelley (1980) has also noticed this and believes it is an important neglected symptom of alopecia areata.

Much grosser changes are seen occasionally. Most nails (finger and toe) are involved. They become rough, opalescent, some are thinned and some thickened (Fig. 5.23). Several will show koilonychia. The changes are identical with those described under the heading of 'severe nail dystrophy' (p. 202). Punctate leukonychia occasionally occurs (Dotz,

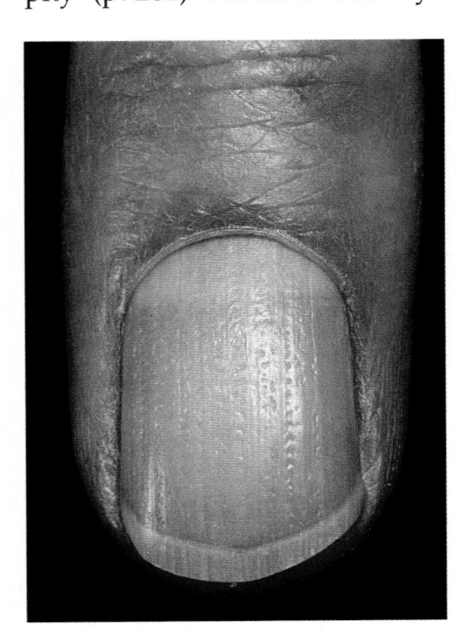

Fig. 5.19
Alopecia areata—uniform pitting

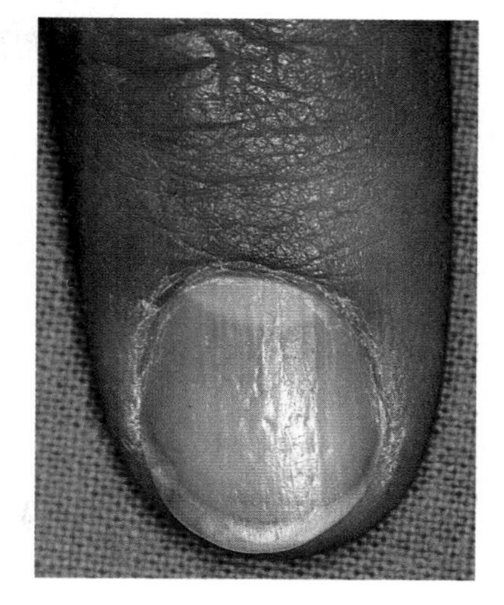

Fig. 5.20 Alopecia areata—uniform pitting

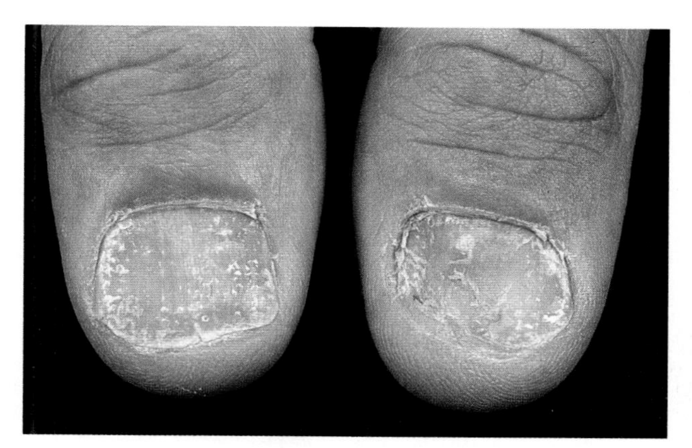

Fig. 5.21 Alopecia areata—pitting and distortion of nail plate

Leiber and Vogt, 1985) as can onycholysis and onychomadesis. Treatment has little effect on the process, although topical steroids are worth trying.

Nail changes are most often seen in association with severe alopecia (Fig. 5.24), but not always so, and occasionally the nail changes predominate. The changes may be observed to appear following the onset of alopecia but once established may persist after the hair fall has ceased. We have seen patients referred on account of their nail dystrophy who have developed alopecia areata months later. Some cases of

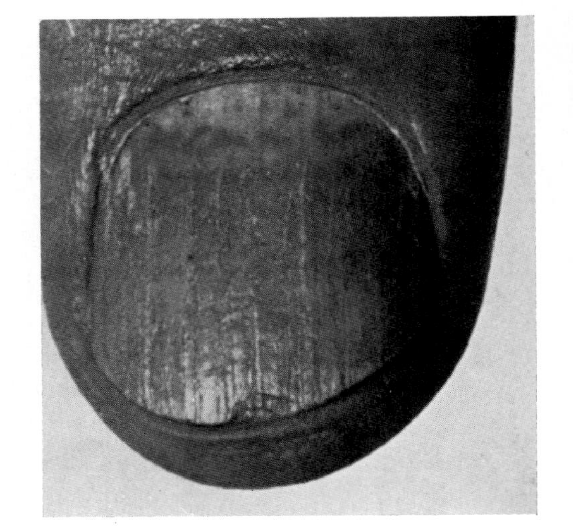

Fig. 5.22 Alopecia areata (universalis) showing mottling in halfmoon area

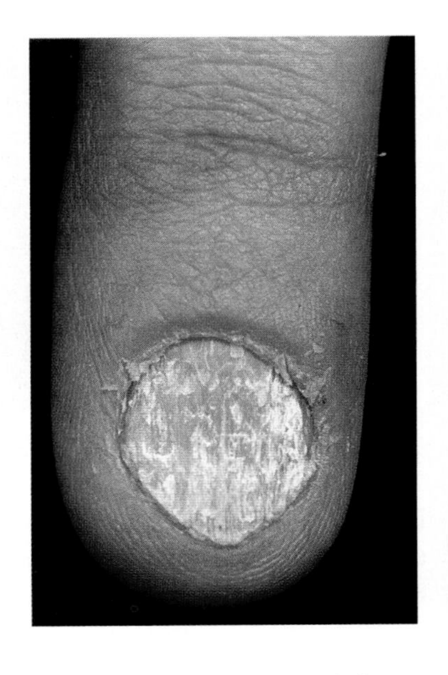

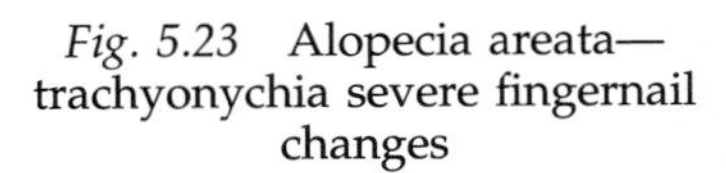

Fig. 5.23 Alopecia areata—trachyonychia severe fingernail changes

nail pitting without alopecia must have the same aetiology. Treatment has little effect on the process although topical steroids are worth trying.

Two cases associated with total vitiligo were described by Demis and Weiner (1963).

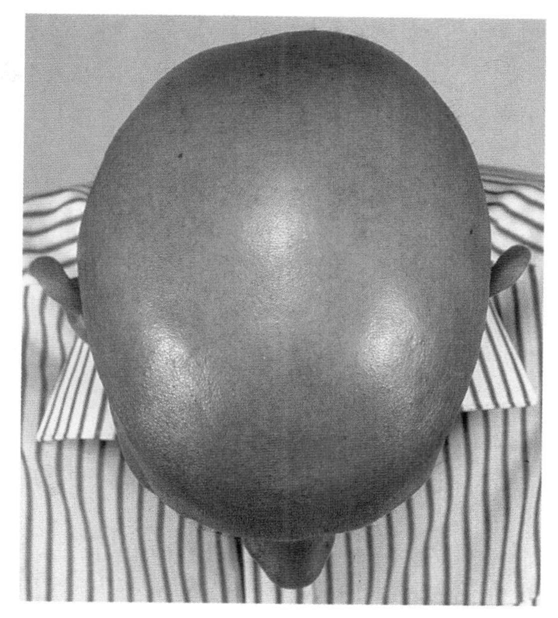

Fig. 5.24 Alopecia areata (totalis)

Pityriasis rubra pilaris

In this disease the nail changes are frequently seen and may closely simulate the grosser changes of psoriasis with thickening of the nail plate and the nail bed (Fig. 5.25). Sonnex *et al.* (1986) found onycholysis in 37% and subungual hyperkeratosis, discoloration, nail plate thickening and splinter haemorrhages in over 70% of 24 patients with adult type I pityriasis rubia pilaris. On other occasions cross ridging may occur as in dermatitis.

Reiter's syndrome

When the skin is involved in this condition the lesions are scaly or crusted and described as keratoderma. When this occurs, and it is rather rare, the nails are likely to be involved

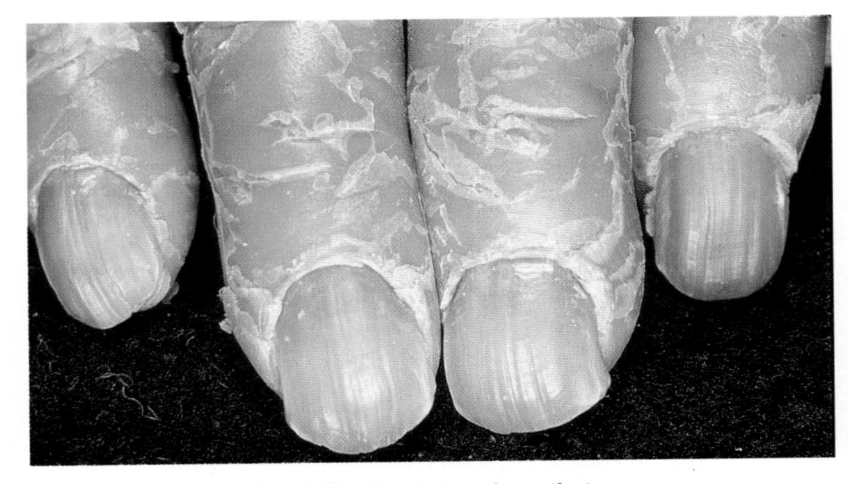

Fig. 5.25 Pityriasis rubra pilaris

and then show changes which are similar to the grosser changes of psoriasis. The nails may also be displaced by the development of hyperkeratosis of the nail bed (Fig. 5.26). Deep pits or even punched-out areas are seen occasionally (Fig. 5.27).

Reiter's disease is one of the conditions associated with HLA B27 inheritance. Pajarre and Kero (1977) describe a case where nail changes were the first manifestation of this inheritance. The patient was a boy of 6; his father suffered from chronic arthritis and recurrent anterior uveitis. Both the boy and his father had HLA combinations of A2 and B27.

Dijkstra (1980) described a case with severe nail changes which rapidly returned to normal after treatment with tetracycline. Another patient with etretinate nail involvement resolved after 1 month's treatment with methotrexate (Ingram and Scher, 1985).

Radiodermatitis

Many years after an excessive dose of X-ray locally, either therapeutic or accidental (for instance, in dental surgeons and radiologists), the nails may become rough and discoloured. The tell-tale telangiectasia and atrophy of the sur-

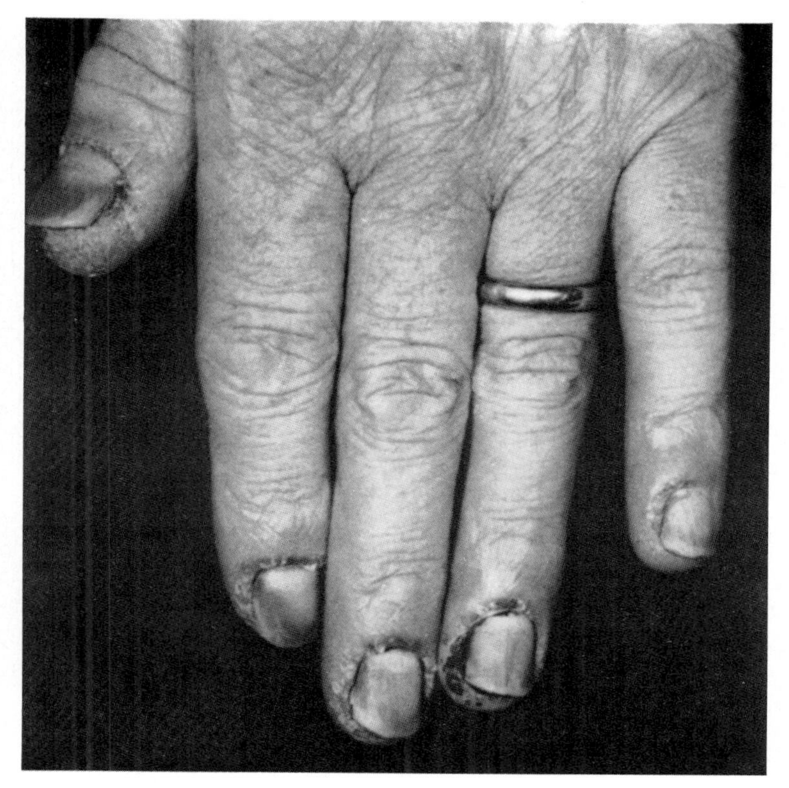

Fig. 5.26 Reiter's syndrome—hyperkeratosis around and under nail

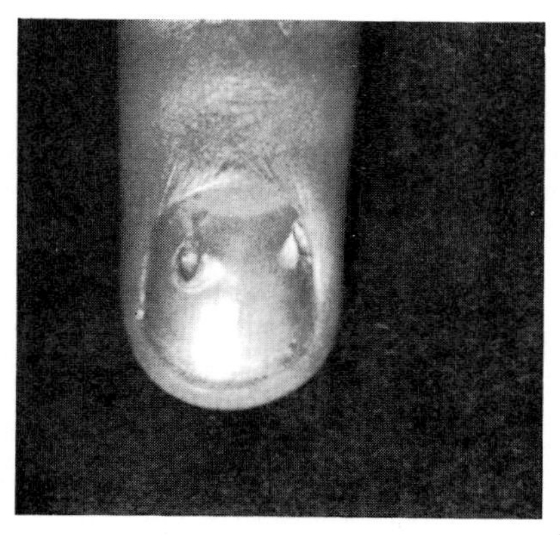

Fig. 5.27 Reiter's syndrome—punched out area of nail plate

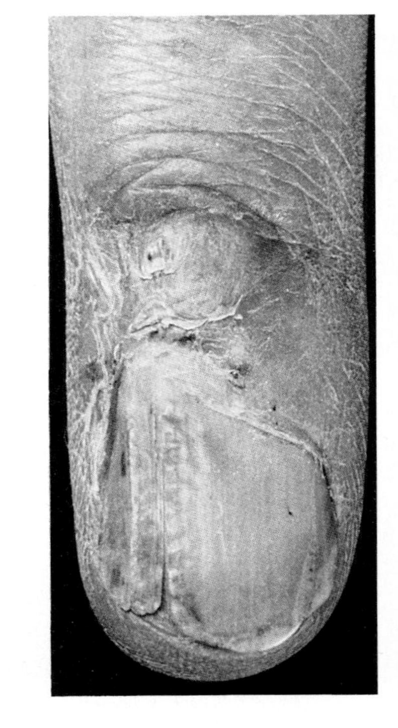

Fig. 5.28 Radiodermatitis following treatment of a periungual wart

rounding soft tissues leave no doubt about the diagnosis. The excess X-ray may result from a single application, such as for treatment of a periungual wart (Fig. 5.28) or more often from repeated small doses over a period of months or years.

Pemphigus

Various dystrophic changes may occur if bullae of pemphigus vulgaris involve the fingertips. In pemphigus foliaceus cross-ridging may occur and shedding of the nails has been reported.

Epidermolysis bullosa dystrophica

There are several varieties of this rare disorder. Permanent loss (Fig. 5.29) of one or more nails is comparatively common and occurs before the patients reach adult life. It is usually impossible to say at what age the nail was actually lost but blistering in the neighbourhood of the nail probably precedes the scarring. On other occasions the affected nails may be only partly destroyed.

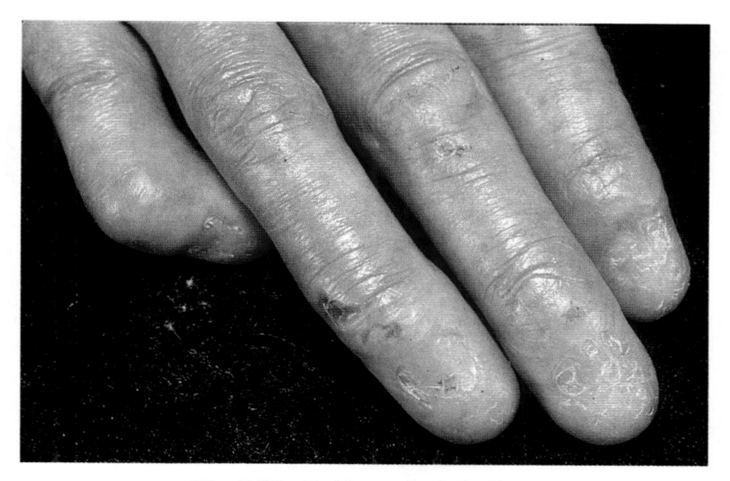

Fig. 5.29 Epidermolysis bullosa

Acanthosis nigricans

In this rare disease the nails may become thickened and discoloured (Fig. 5.30).

Sarcoidosis (Figs 5.31, 5.32)

Sarcoidosis of the lupus pernio type often affects the digits of fingers or toes. If the damage is situated close to the nail, the latter may be deformed in various ways. It may become thickened and very irregular (Fig. 5.33), it may become defective especially near the tip, or it may be lost altogether. X-ray will often show that the underlying bone has been damaged (Fig. 5.34). Pterygium formation is also recorded (Kalb and Grossman, 1985).

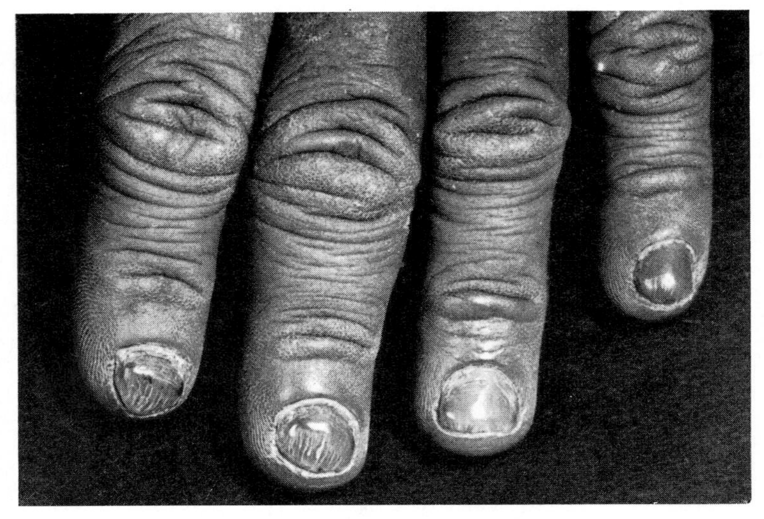

Fig. 5.30 Acanthosis nigricans

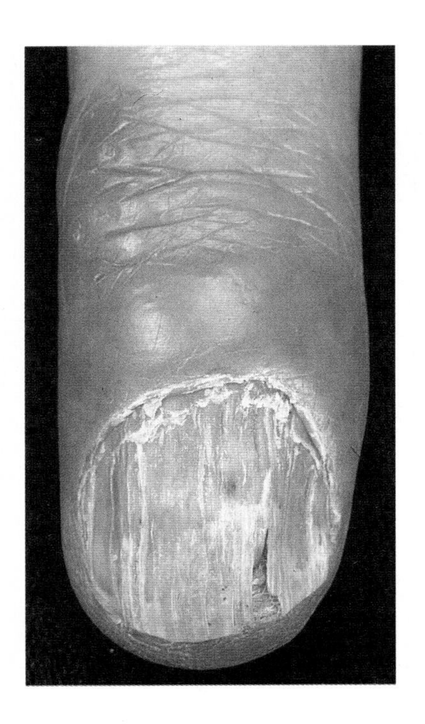

Fig. 5.31 Sarcoidosis

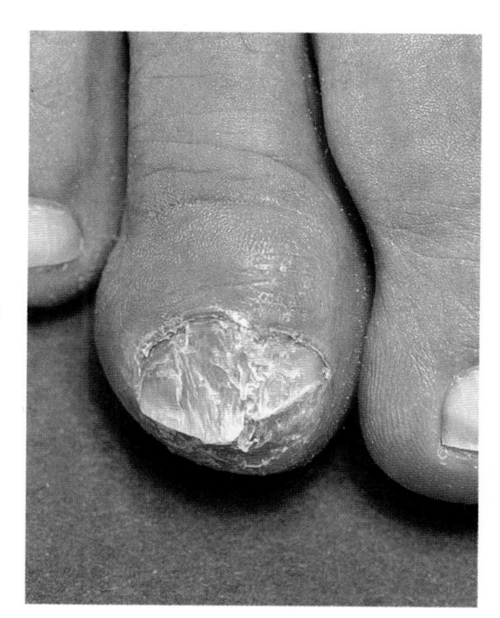

Fig. 5.32 Sarcoidosis—lupus pernio

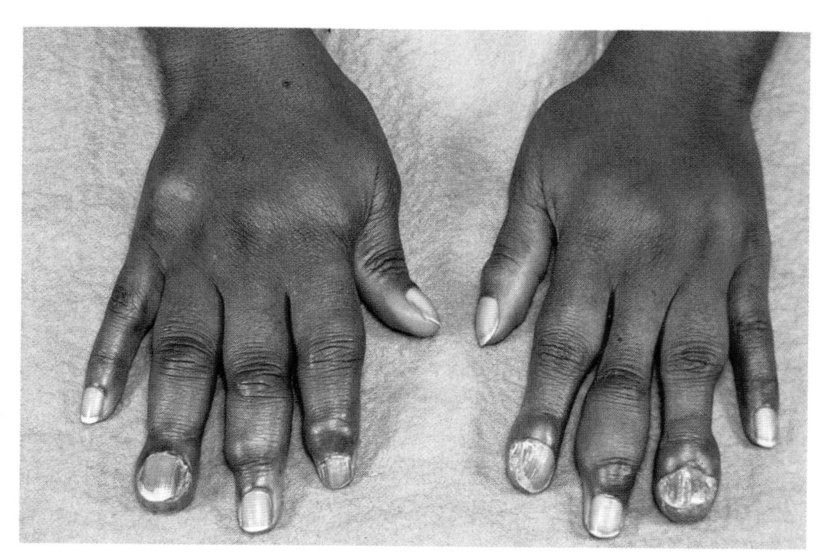

Fig. 5.33 Sarcoidosis

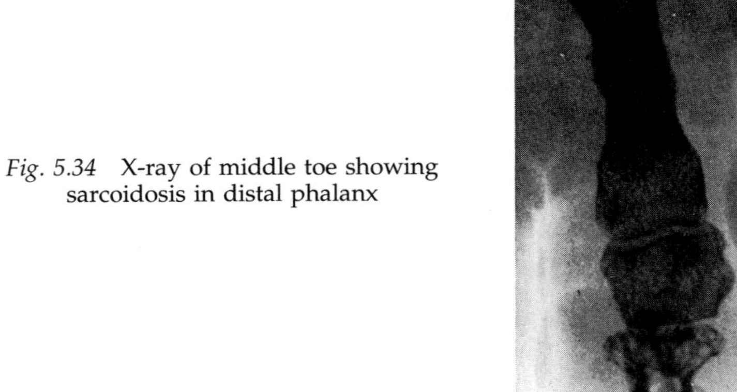

Fig. 5.34 X-ray of middle toe showing sarcoidosis in distal phalanx

Porokeratosis (mibelli)

The nails are occasionally damaged in this rare disorder. Figure 5.35 shows splitting, ridging and partial destruction of three nails, changes which closely resemble those of impaired peripheral circulation.

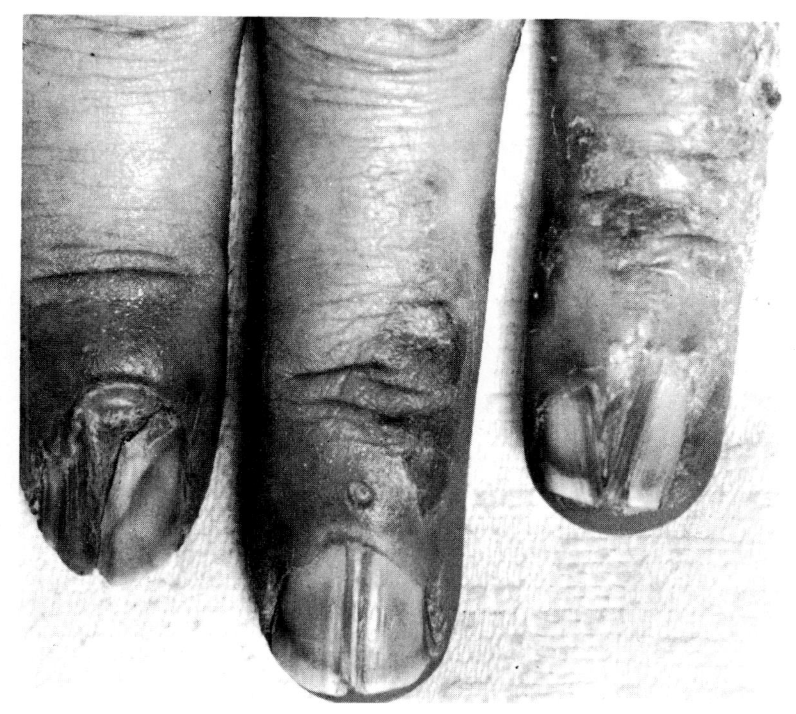

Fig. 5.35 Porokeratosis of Mibelli

References

Baran, R, Dupré, A, Lavret, P and Puissant, A (1979) Le lichen striatus onychodystrophique. *Ann. Derm. Venereol.* (*Paris*) **106** 885

Burge, S M, Wilkinson, J D and Miller, A J, *et al.* (1981) The efficacy of an aromatic retinoid, Tigason (etretinate), in the treatment of Darier's disease. *Brit. J. Derm.* **104** 675

Burgoon, C F Jr. and Kostrazewa, R M (1969) Lichen planus limited to the nails. *Arch. Derm.* **100** 371

Cornelius, C E III and Shelley, W B (1967) Permanent anonychia due to lichen planus. *Arch. Derm.* **96** 434

Cram, D L, Kierland, R R and Winkelmann, R K (1966) Ulcerative lichen planus of the feet. *Arch. Derm.* **93** 692

Degos, R and Schnitzler, L (1967) Lichen erosive des Orteils. *Ann. Derm. Syph.* (*Paris*) **94** 241

Demis, D J and Weiner, M R (1963) Alopecia universalis, onychodystrophy and total vitiligo. *Arch. Derm.* **88** 195

Dijkstra, J H E (1980) Nail involvement in Reiter's disease. *Brit. J. Derm.* **102** 480

Dotz, W I, Lieber, C D and Vogt, P J. (1985) Leuconychia punctate and pitted nails in alopecia areata. *Arch. Derm.* **121** 1452

Fisher, A A. (1986) *Contact Dermatitis*, 3rd ed. Philadelphia: Lea and Febiger

Ganor, S (1977) Diseases sometimes associated with psoriasis. 11 Alopecia areata. *Dermatologica* **154** 338

Ingram, G J and Scher, R K (1985) Reiter's Syndrome with nail involvement. Is It psoriasis? *Cutis* **36** 37

Kalb, R E and Grossman, M E. (1985) Pterygium formation due to sarcoidosis. *Arch. Derm.* **121** 276

Kaufman, J P (1974) Lichen striatus with nail involvement. *Cutis* **14** 232

Marks, R and Samman, P D (1972) Isolated nail dystrophy due to lichen planus. *Trans. St John's Hosp. Derm Soc.* **58** 93

Niren, N M, Waldman, G D and Barsky, S (1981) Lichen striatus with onychodystrophy. *Cutis* **27** 610

Pajarre, R and Kero, M (1977) Nail changes as first manifestation of HLA B27 inheritance. *Dermatologica* **154** 350

Ronchese, F (1965) The nail in Darier's disease. *Arch. Derm.* **91** 617

Rubisz Brzerzinska, J and Seferowicz, E (1974) Studies on the incidence of lesions in the nail plates in alopecia areata (Polish). *Przegal Derm.* **61** 147

Samman, P D (1961) The nails in lichen planus. *Brit. J. Derm.* **73** 288

Savin, J A and Samman, P D (1970) The nail in Darier's disease. *Med. Biol. Illus.* **20** 85

Scher, R K, Fischbein, R and Ackerman, A B (1978) 20 Nail dystrophy. A variant of lichen planus. *Arch. Derm.* **114** 612

Schubert, H (1966) Nagelveranderungen bei Morbus Darier. *Z. Haut-und Gesch.* **41** 239

Shelley, W B (1972) Onycholysis due to topical 5 fluorouracil. *Acta Derm. Venereol. (Stock).* **52** 320

Shelley, W B (1980) The spotted lunula. A neglected sign associated with alopecia areata. *J. Amer. Acad. Derm.* **2** 385

Sonnex, T S, Dawber, R P R, Zachary, C B, *et al.* (1986) The nails in adult type I pityriasis rubra pilaris. *J. Amer. Acad. Derm.* **15** 956

Zaias, N (1970) The nail in lichen planus. *Arch. Derm.* **101** 264

Zaias, N (1980) *The Nail in Health and Disease*. New York: Spectrum

Zaias, N and Ackerman, A B (1973) The nail in Darier-White disease. *Arch. Derm.* **107** 193

6

Miscellaneous acquired nail disorders

P. D. Samman and D. A. Fenton

Onycholysis (idiopathic)

Onycholysis as a symptom is mentioned on p. 25. There are many known causes but when they have been excluded many cases remain where no cause can be found.

Spontaneous onycholysis is common and can be very troublesome. The loosened nail is unsightly and dirt which collects beneath it is difficult to remove. In the early stages the condition is painless but the nail loses its value as an aid in the picking up of small objects. The condition is almost always confined to women and is seen especially in persons who like to keep their nails long so that minor trauma may play a part in aetiology. Patients often notice that the affected nails grow faster than their normal nails and measurements have confirmed this (Dawber, Samman and Bottoms, 1971). The reason for the increased growth rate is not yet known.

One or several nails may be involved and usually only part of the nail is separated (Fig. 6.1), but once loosened the nail is subjected to repeated minor traumata which may cause extension of the involved area and is accompanied by pain. The nail bed quickly becomes contaminated by bacteria or yeasts and there may be pus formation but often the infection is asymptomatic. *Pseudomonas aeruginosa* is a

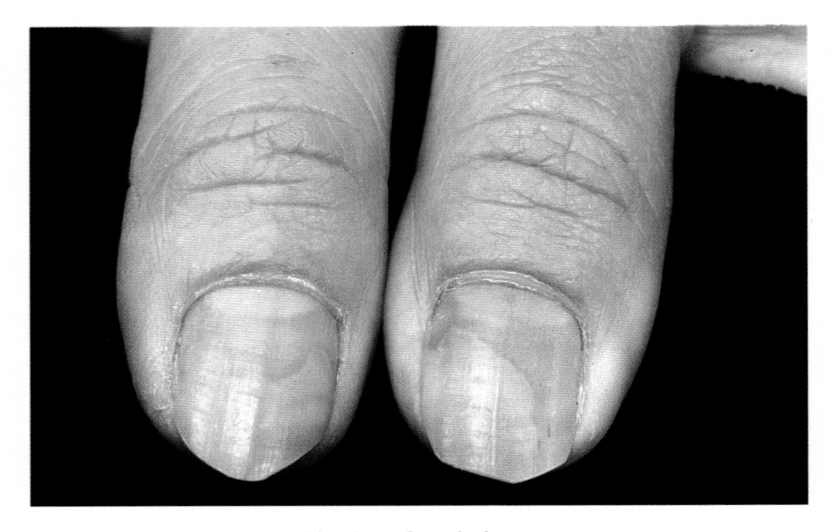

Fig. 6.1 Onycholysis

common contaminant and this will produce a characteristic coloration of the nail plate which may be green, blue or black (Chernosky and Dukes, 1963).

The condition is a very stubborn one, and if not corrected the exposed nail bed becomes covered with keratin very similar to that of the fingertip; when this happens, reattachment of the nail is very unlikely to occur.

The secondary infection is probably the main reason for the failure of the nail to reattach itself in the early stages. Ray (1963) recommends treatment of this by cutting away the loosened nail with sharp pointed nail clippers followed by the application of a 15% solution of sulphacetamide in 50% spirit to the nail bed. This is repeated daily whilst the nail has a chance to grow forward and reattach itself as it does so. Sulphacetamide 15% is bactericidal to all contaminants and also prevents the growth of fungi and yeasts. Wilson (1965) recommended 4% thymol in chloroform as a means of preventing infection and maceration of the nail bed. The author has found that some patients cannot tolerate 4% thymol and prefers 2% in chloroform. Both these methods are useful but neither is successful in every case. Sulphacetamide is applied with a brush, but the thymol solution should be applied with cotton wool on an orange stick.

Dystrophia mediana canaliformis (median nail dystrophy) (Fig. 6.2)

This is an uncommon condition of unknown aetiology first described by Heller (1928). It consists of a split or canal in the nail plate and is usually just off centre. Any finger nail may be involved but more often the thumb nails. The split starts at the cuticle and progresses to the free edge. There are usually a few feathery cracks extending laterally from the split towards, but not reaching, the edges of the nail. This has been likened to an inverted fir tree. After a period of months or years, the nail returns to normal in most cases but relapse may occur (Fig. 6.3). On healing, a ridge normally replaces the split. It is apparent that there is some temporary damage to the nail matrix and as most cases seem to have large half moons, so that a larger part of the matrix is unprotected by the dorsal nail fold than usual, the damage may be of a traumatic nature. A few cases give a definite history of trauma. Familial cases have been recorded (Seller, 1974). Sutton (1965) described a case on a toe nail in which a flabby filament of fleshy tissue was present in the canal. He referred the term 'solenonychia' for this deformity.

Van Duk (1978) described a number of cases, which are all slightly different, but which he believes are variants of the one process. He also gives a good bibliography of the condition.

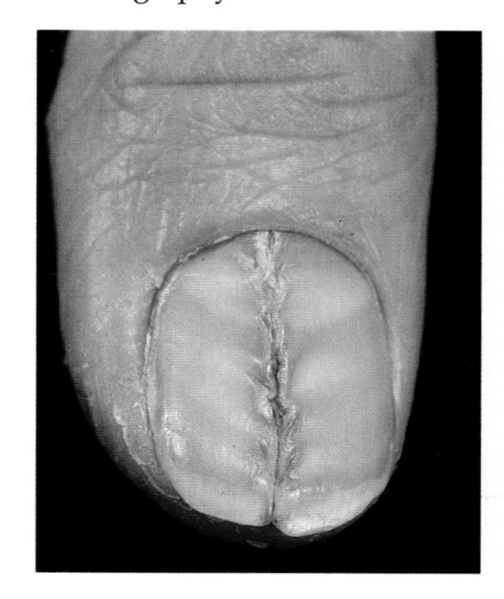

Fig. 6.2 Median nail dystrophy

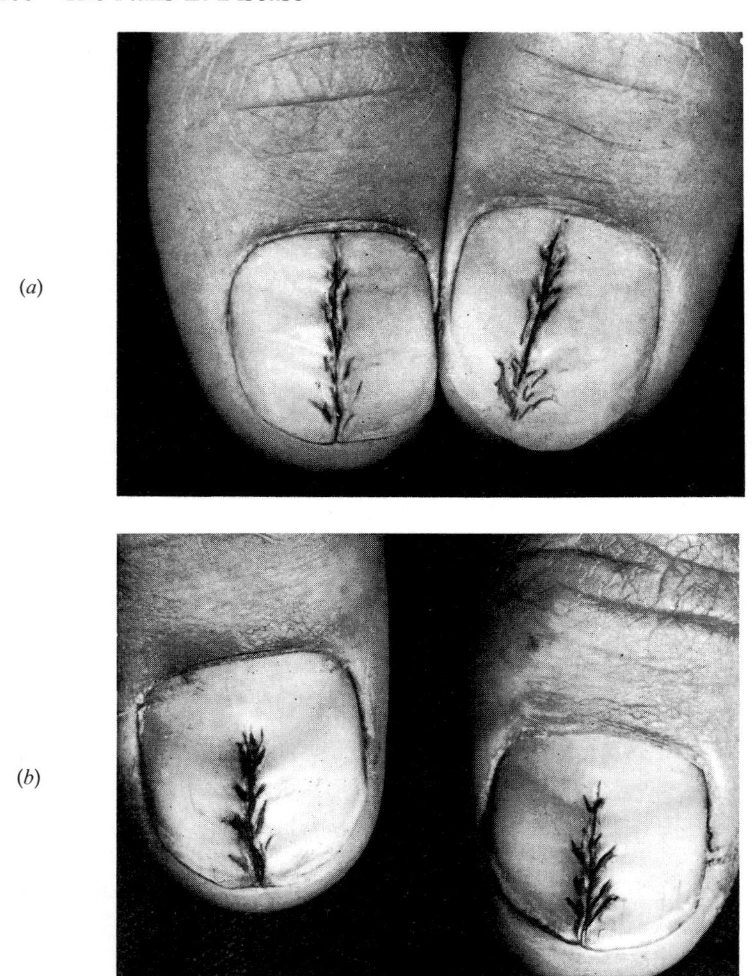

Fig. 6.3 (a) Dystrophia mediana canaliformis (*b*) Same, two months later (*c*) Same, another two months later showing spontaneous improvement

Diagnosis is generally obvious. A split as a result of definite trauma must be excluded as also must repeated trauma due to a habit tic and to splits as seen in the nail patella syndrome.

Treatment is usually unnecessary but protection from trauma is advised. The nail should be kept short to reduce the disability produced by a nail split into halves.

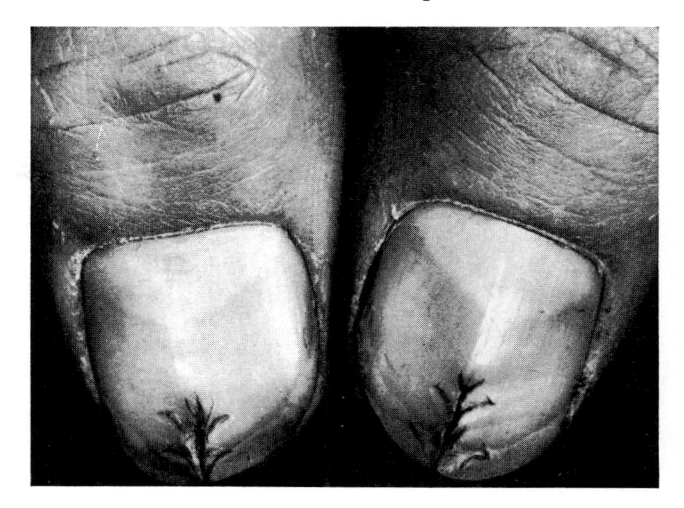

(c)

Leukonychia

This term is used to imply whitening of the nail plate itself. It may be congenital or acquired, partial or complete. The rare congenital leukonychia totalis is described on p. 197. Partial leukonychia is very common and may be punctate (Fig. 6.4) or striate (Figs. 6.5, 6.6). It may occasionally be the result of illness, for example, Mees' stripes in chronic arsenical poisoning, and has been described in association with many other diseases (Albright and Wheeler, 1964). In the great majority of punctate cases, however, which are extremely common, no cause can be found. Mitchell (1953) made an interesting study of his own nails over a period of a year and showed that some white spots appeared near the cuticle but others were on other parts of the nail. Some disappeared before they reached the free edge and some increased in size after they had been formed.

In striate leukonychia a traumatic element is present in some cases and in particular overzealous manicuring. The condition will resolve if less active manicure is used. There is no very satisfactory explanation for the whiteness but it may be due to incomplete keratinisation so that nuclei or nuclear debris are retained in the nail plate.

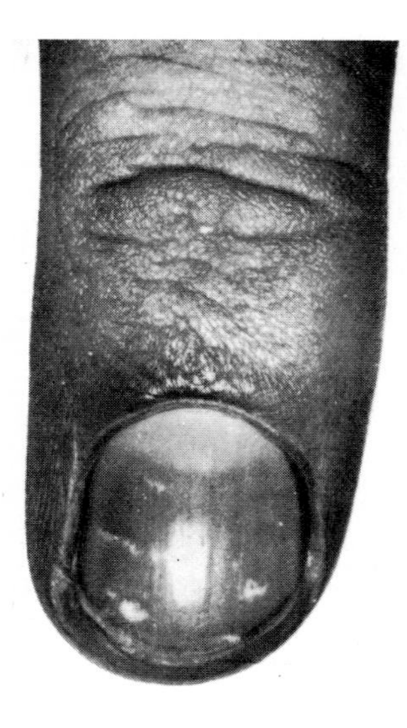

Fig. 6.4 Leukonychia punctata

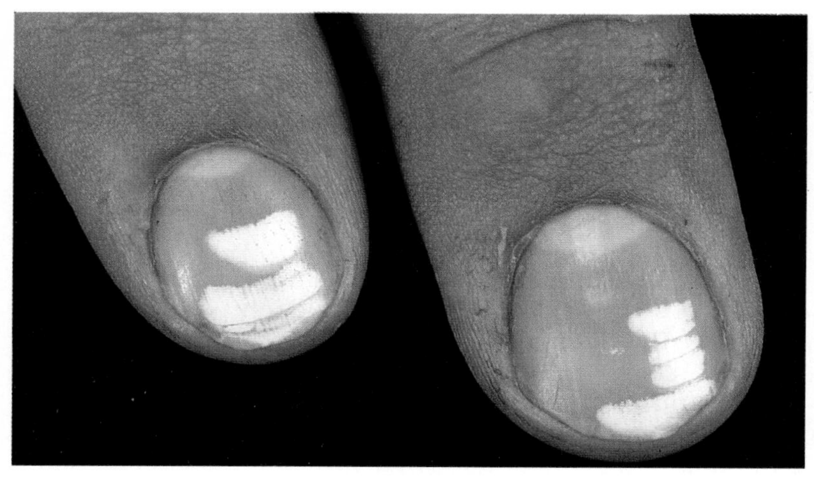

Fig. 6.5 Leukonychia striata

Leukonychia must be distinguished from whitening due to other causes, such as fungal infection of the nail plate and whiteness of the nail bed in hypoalbuminaemia.

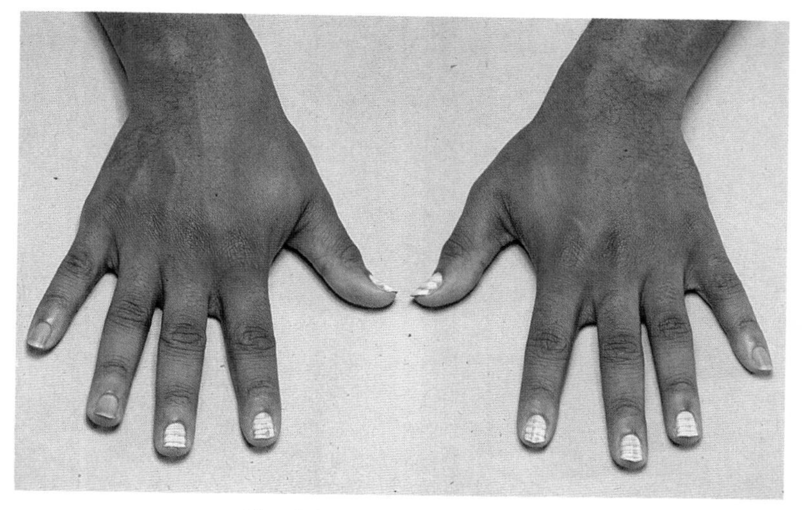

Fig. 6.6 Leukonychia striata

Leukonychia striata longitudinalis

Under this title, Higashi, Sugai and Yamamoto (1971) described the occurrence in two patients of a white streak extending from cuticle to free margin and lasting for several years. In one case the white streak was attributed to the presence of abnormal cornified cells in the nail plate accompanied by parakeratotic hyperplasia of the nail bed epidermis and in the other to parakeratotic hyperplasia of the nail bed epidermis only. The condition was thought to be due to naevoid changes in the distal nail matrix below the white streak.

It would be difficult to differentiate this condition from white streaks in the nails in Darier's disease unless other evidence of that condition was present.

Parakeratosis pustulosa (Figs. 6.7, 6.8, 6.9)

Under this heading Hjorth and Thomsen (1967) described a disorder confined to young children and especially girls. The lesions begin close to the free margin of the nail, and in about 25% of cases a few isolated pustules or vesicles can be seen in the initial phase. These quickly clear and eczematoid changes

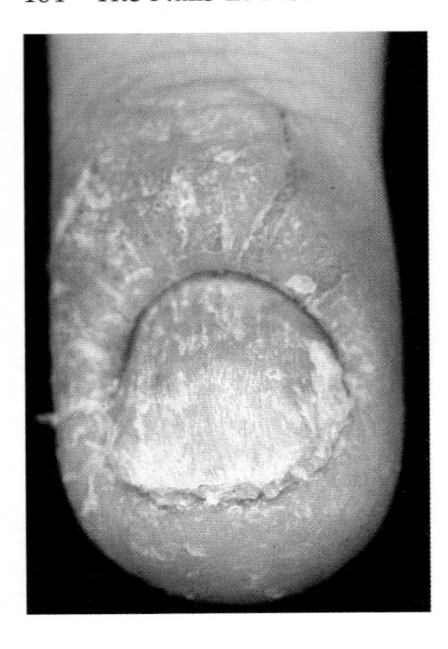

Fig. 6.7 Parakeratosis pustulata

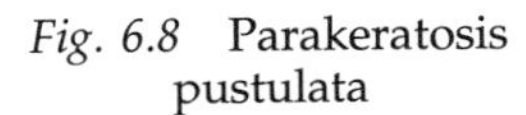

Fig. 6.8 Parakeratosis pustulata

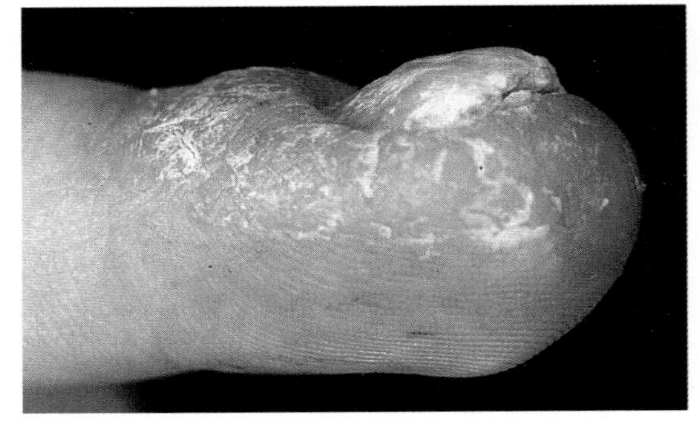

cover the skin immediately adjacent to the free margin of the nail. The changes may extend to the dorsal nail fold or to the sides of finger or toe. The most striking and characteristic changes result from hyperkeratosis under the free margin of the nail which rarely extends more than 1–2 mm into the nail bed. The nail itself is lifted and deformed and sometimes thickened. There may be pitting and rarely cross-ridging. The condition is more common on the hands and is usually limited to one digit, occasionally two, rarely more. On the hands the thumb and index finger are most often affected

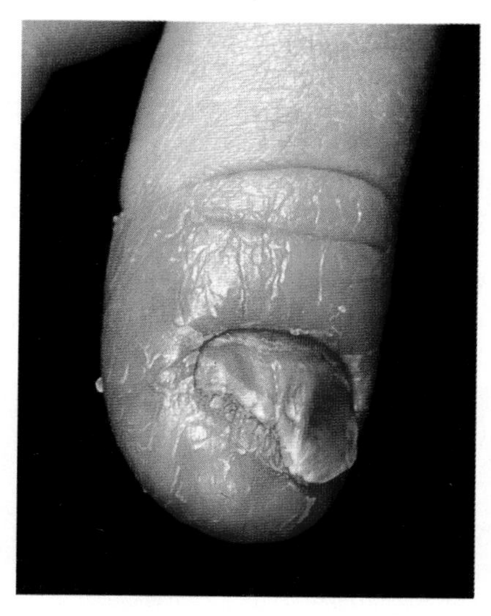

Fig. 6.9 Parakeratosis pustulata

and on the feet, the great toes. The condition lasts a long time—often for a number of years—and may recur after apparent cure and may then affect a different digit. It does not, however, extend into adult life.

The author has seen a number of cases which would conform to this description. The changes are at times very like psoriasis but Hjorth and Thomsen consider the condition to be an independent eczematoid eruption. Dulanto, Armigo-Moreno and Camacho-Martinez (1974) and Botela *et al.* (1973) do not agree with this and suggest that it may be due to psoriasis, pustular psoriasis or eczema. Dulanto *et al.* give the histological findings in one case and they are indefinite.

Idiopathic atrophy of the nails

This is an uncommon condition. The nails are normal at birth but after a few years one or more nails become deformed. The condition is progressive for a time, then becomes stationary, but any damage is permanent. The changes vary from excessive ridging and opacity to pterygium formation and on some digits to total loss of the nail with scarring (Fig. 6.10). Finger nails are more often affected than toe nails.

Although some patients appear to have poor peripheral circulation, this does not seem to be an important feature and the complete absence of pain or discomfort rules out an inflammatory process such as lichen planus. There are no skin lesions elsewhere (Samman, 1969). In one black family two sisters showed lesions very similar to one another. Epidermolysis bullosa must be considered.

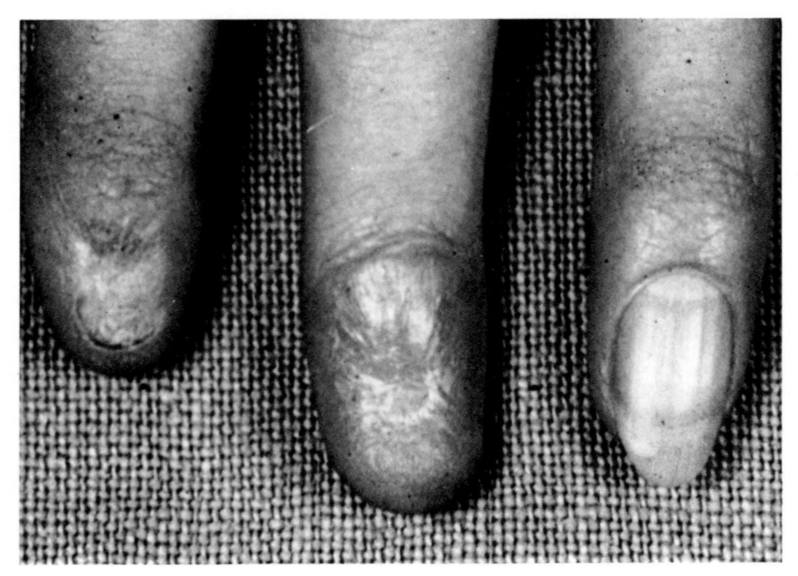

Fig. 6.10 Idiopathic atrophy—loss with scarring

Pterygium inversum unguis

Under this heading Caputo and Prandi (1973) described a patient who had an acquired abnormality in which the distal part of the nail bed remained adherent to the ventral surface of the nail plate, thus eliminating the distal groove. It involved several fingers and there was no alteration of the nail plate. The patient suffered pain and bleeding if she attempted to cut the nails.

A few similar reports have appeared subsequently. The author has seen a number of cases (Fig. 6.11) including one where two toes were affected.

Christophers (1975) describes under the heading of familial subungual pterygium a mother and daughter who each had a condition of a similar nature which was also painful. This type of change is not infrequently seen in patients with scleroderma of the progressive type, the result of local soft tissue atrophy.

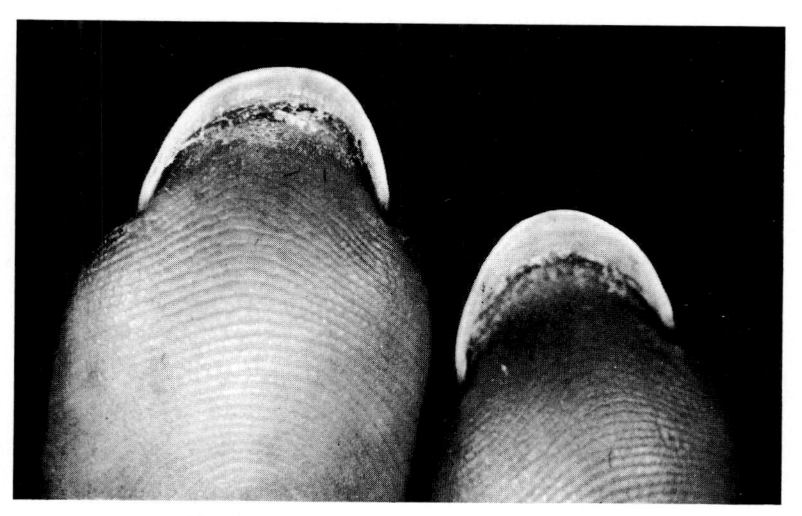

Fig. 6.11 Pterygium inversum unguis

Brittle nails

As mentioned under symptomatology, brittle nails are very common and generally no cause can be found. The character of a nail varies considerably according to its water content. A normal nail contains about 18% water vapour. If this is greatly increased, for example, after prolonged immersion in water, the nail becomes very soft. Alternatively, if it is considerably reduced the nail becomes brittle. This excess loss is liable to occur in a dry atmosphere and is equivalent to skin chapping. It is also liable to occur more rapidly if the nail is thin and if the nail is kept long so that there is more than the usual amount exposed to the atmosphere on upper and lower surfaces. It is not known how much of the moisture content of nail keratin is derived from the atmosphere and how much from the underlying soft tissues. Close attachment to the nail bed with the nails cut short to reduce the surface area exposed to the atmosphere will certainly restrict the amount of loss in a dry atmosphere. The brittleness is due to a lowered water content of the nail but the splitting which results from the brittleness is probably partly due to repeated increase and decrease of water content so that the nail changes from soft to brittle frequently during the course of a day.

Treatment of brittle nails must be symptomatic. Avoidance of a very dry atmosphere and of frequent immersion of the hands in water is recommended. The nails should be kept trimmed as short as possible and the use of hand cream at night, especially one containing glycerin, may be helpful, for example, equal parts of 2% salicyclic acid ointment and glycerin of starch. This should be applied regularly all over the fingertips. The use of nail varnish is not contraindicated.

Damage caused by weed killers

Samman and Johnstone (1969) recorded cases of damage to finger nails resulting from contact with concentrated solutions of paraquat and diquat. The material must have penetrated to the nail matrix and interfered with the growth of the nails. The changes ranged from white or brown bands across the base of the nails with softening of the nail plate to permanent loss of one nail (Figs. 6.12, 6.13). Hearn and Keir (1971) have recorded similar damage following gross contamination with diluted solutions.

It seems probable that other chemicals which interfere with keratinisation could produce a similar deformity if allowed to enter the posterior nail fold. The author has seen a patient with severe damage from hydrofluoric acid (Fig. 6.14) (Samman, 1977).

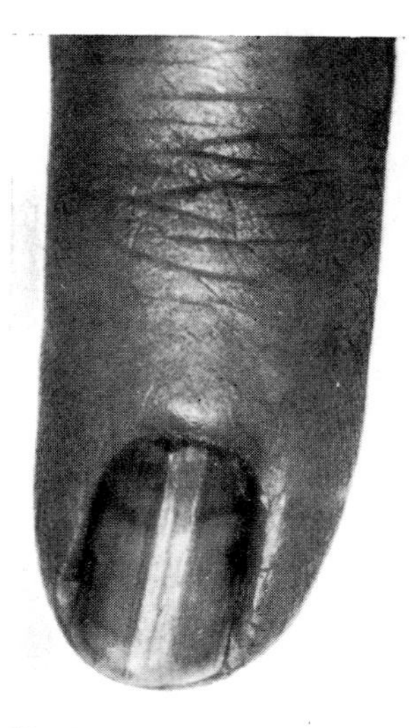

Fig. 6.12 Damage caused by weed killers

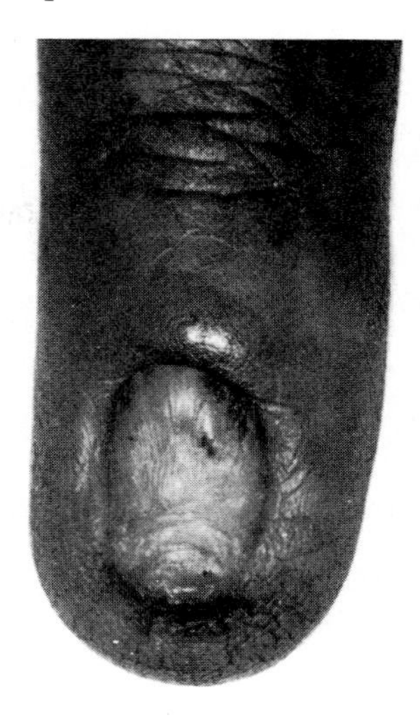

Fig. 6.13 Damage caused by weed killers

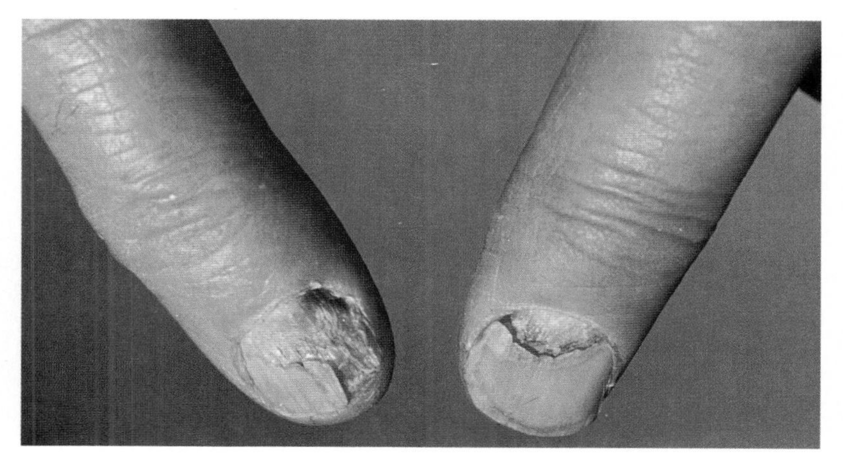

Fig. 6.14 Damage to nails due to contact with dilute hydrofluoric acid

References

Albright, S D and Wheeler, C E (1964) Leukonychia. *Arch. Derm.* **90** 392

Botela, R, Mascaro, J M, Martinez, C and Albero, F (1973) La parakeratosis pustulosa. *Acta. Derm. Syph.* **64** 579

Caputo, M E and Prandi, G (1973) Pterygium inversum unguis. *Arch. Derm.* **108** 817

Chernosky, M E and Dukes, C D (1963) Green nails. Importance of *Pseudomonas aeruginosa* in onychia. *Arch. Derm.* **88** 548

Christophers, E (1975) Familial subungual pterygium. *Der Hautarzt* **26** 543

Dawber, R P R, Samman, P D and Bottoms, E (1971) Finger nail growth in idiopathic and psoriatic onycholysis. *Brit. J. Derm.* **85** 558

Dulanto, F de, Armigo-Moreno and Camacho-Martinez, F (1974) Parakeratosis pustulose: histological findings. *Acta Dermatovenereol. (Stock.)* **54** 365

Hearn, C E D and Keir, W (1971) Nail damage in spray operators exposed to paraquat. *Brit. J. Indust. Med.* **28** 399

Heller, J (1928) Dystrophia unguium mediana canaliformis. *Derm. Z* **51** 416

Higashi, N, Sugai, T and Yamamoto, T (1971) Leukonychia striata longitudinales. *Arch. Derm.* **104** 192

Hjorth, N and Thomsen, K (1967) Parakeratosis pustulosa. *Brit. J. Derm.* **79** 527

Mitchell, J C (1953) A clinical study of leukonychia. *Brit. J. Derm.* **65** 121

Ray, L (1963) Onycholysis. *Arch. Derm.* **88** 181

Samman, P D (1969) Idiopathic atrophy of the nails. *Brit. J. Derm.* **81** 746

Samman, P D (1977) Nail disorders caused by external influences. *J. Soc. Cosmet. Chem.* **28** 351

Samman, P D and Johnstone, E N M (1969) Nail damage associated with handling of paraquat and diquat. *Brit. Med. J.* **1** 818

Seller, H (1974) Dystrophia unguis mediana canaliformis: familial occurrence. *Der Hautarzt* **25** 456

Sutton, R L Jr (1965) Solenonychia. *Sth. Med. J. (Nashville)* **58** 1143

Van Duk (1978) Dystrophia unguium mediana canaliformis. *Dermatologica* **156** 358

Wilson, J W (1965) Paronychia and onycholysis. Etiology and therapy. *Arch. Derm.* **92** 726

7

Nail disorders associated with general medical conditions

D. A. Fenton

Koilonychia

In this condition loss of the normal contour occurs so that the nail becomes flat (platonychia) (Fig. 7.1) or concave (spoon-shaped-koilonychia) (Fig. 7.2). It is a common finding in infants, affecting both fingers and toe nails but usually soon becomes corrected. Sometimes it occurs as a developmental anomaly (Hellier, 1950) where it is inherited as an autosomal dominant gene (Handa *et al.*, 1960) although expression may be incomplete in certain cases.

It is, however, the classical nail disorder of iron-deficiency anaemia. Although usually confined to the fingers in anaemia, it may occur on the toe nails. It is a common manifestation of the Plummer–Vinson syndrome in association with dysphagia and glossitis. Cystine deficiency has been demonstrated in affected nails (Jalili and Al-Kassab, 1959), but this has not been confirmed.

Koilonychia is due to thinning and softening of the nail plate. It can occur at times in the presence of low iron stores without anaemia (Beutler, 1964; Comaish, 1965). It is also seen in haemachromatosis, Raynaud's syndrome and porphyria. The separated halves of nails affected by pterygium

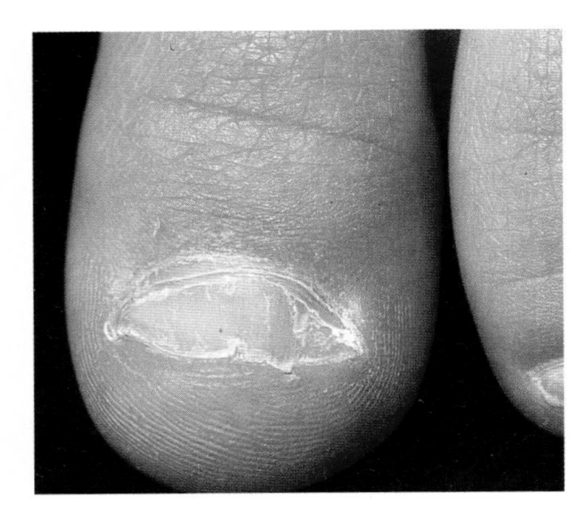

Fig. 7.1 Platonychia

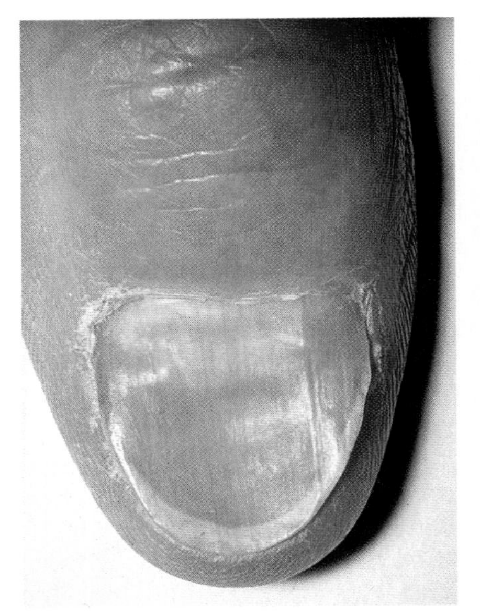

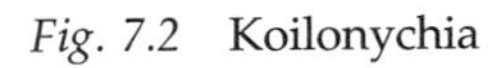

Fig. 7.2 Koilonychia

formation may be spoon-shaped, as may the two halves of split nails in the nail-patella syndrome.

Occasionally it occurs as an occupational disorder, probably as a result of softening with soaps or oils (Fig. 7.3). It is seen in motor mechanics (Dawber, 1974) and on the toes of ricksha boys in South Africa as a result of trauma (Bentley-Phillips and Bayles, 1971). It was also seen with benoxaprofen therapy.

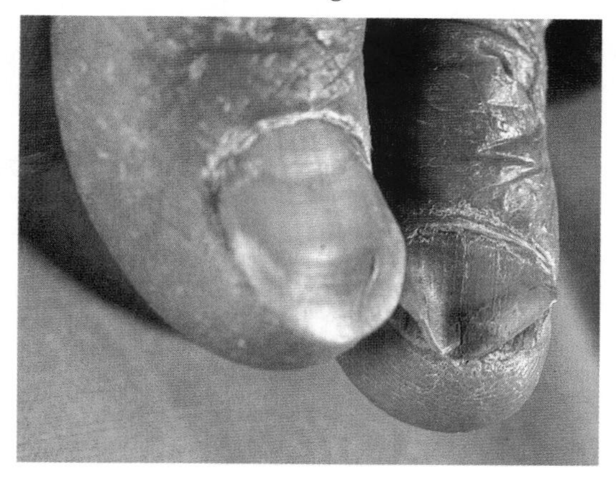

Fig. 7.3 Occupational koilonychia

In iron deficiency with or without anaemia, the administration of iron corrects the deformity.

Clubbing

The earliest change is loss of the normal angle between the nail and the posterior nail fold (Lovibond's angle). Later the distal phalanx becomes enlarged and there may be an increase in the size of the nail (Figs. 7.4, 7.5). Although usually an important physical sign, it is occasionally present from birth without any underlying disease and it may be familial.

Clubbing is classically associated with suppurative lung disease or cyanotic heart disease. A more severe form, known as hypertrophic pulmonary osteoarthropathy, is characterised by periostitis affecting the metacarpals, the two proximal rows of phalanges and distal ulnar and radius, and corresponding bones in the feet and legs. Most of these cases are due to bronchogenic carcinoma and, less commonly, bronchiectasis.

A third extremely rare form, pachydermoperiostosis, is generally considered idiopathic. In addition to clubbing there is a spade-like enlargement of the hands, hyperhidrosis and thickening of the legs, forearms and facial tissues. It mainly affects adolescent males and is self-limiting.

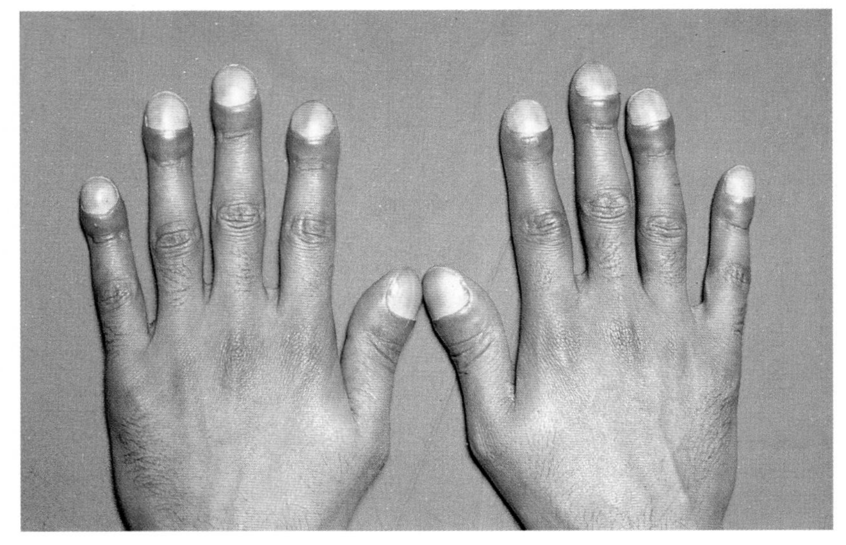

Fig. 7.4 Finger clubbing

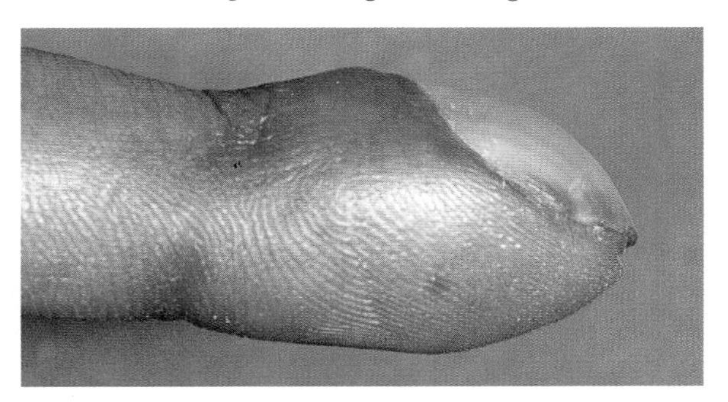

Fig. 7.5 Finger clubbing—lateral view

Clubbing occurs in thyrotoxicosis, and several gastrointestinal disorders including ulcerative colitis, Crohn's disease, tropical sprue and biliary cirrhosis. It has been suggested that it occurs only if the diseased organ is innervated by the vagus nerve (Young, 1966); thus in ulcerative colitis clubbing only occurs if the disease affects part of the colon which is supplied by the vagus.

Arteriography demonstrates abundant blood flow through the digits possibly due to opening up of arteriovenous anastomoses. When clubbing is present mixed arterial and venous blood is shunted past normal lung tissue; Hall (1959) suggests that the substance present in venous blood which is responsible for opening up the arteriovenous anastomosis is reduced ferritin. On oxidation, by passing through normal lung tissue, it becomes inert.

Stone and Maberry (1965) and Stone (1975) put forward an hypothesis to explain the abnormal shapes of nails in clubbing and koilonychia. They suggest that nail formation follows simple structural rules. Nail is much like a sheet of plastic being extruded during the period of keratinisation. They consider that there must be some common mechanism for the formation of clubbed and spoon-shaped nails. The diverse disorders which will produce these changes are more likely to have an effect on connective tissue than on hard keratin.

Nail changes in spooning and clubbing are the result of an angulation of the (principal) matrix secondary to connective tissue changes. Spooning occurs if the distal end of the matrix is relatively low compared with the proximal end and clubbing if the distal end is relatively high compared with the proximal end. In severe anaemia the distal end may be depressed below its normal level due to anoxia and atrophy of the distal connective tissue. In clubbing there is an increase in volume of the distal phalanx due to connective tissue proliferation and at times due to increased vascular flow. This will result in the distal end of the matrix being elevated.

Beau's lines

These are transverse ridges in the nail plate due to a temporary alteration of nail growth rate. The condition is represented by a depression on the surface of all the nails (Figs. 7.6, 7.7). The lines appear from under the cuticle about a month following the initial illness. In severe cases the depression extends completely through the nail plate leading to temporary shedding of the nails (Fig. 7.8) (Beau, 1846).

Acute febrile illnesses and severe disabilities including measles, mumps, pneumonia, myocardial infarction and pulmonary embolism may be responsible.

The lines enable the causative illness to be dated. Similar lines, but only affecting a few nails, may be seen in Raynaud's

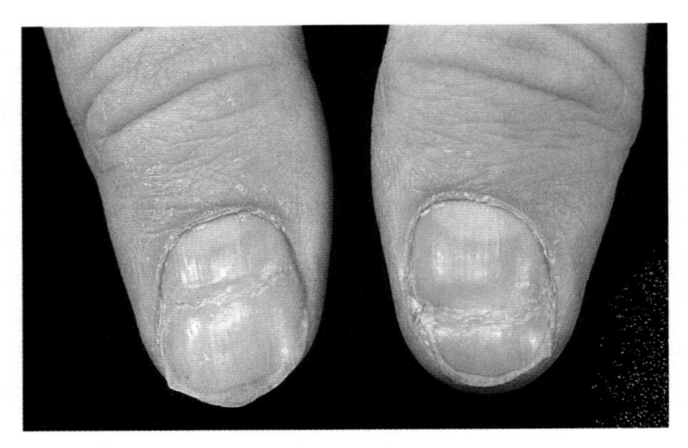

Fig. 7.6 Beau's lines

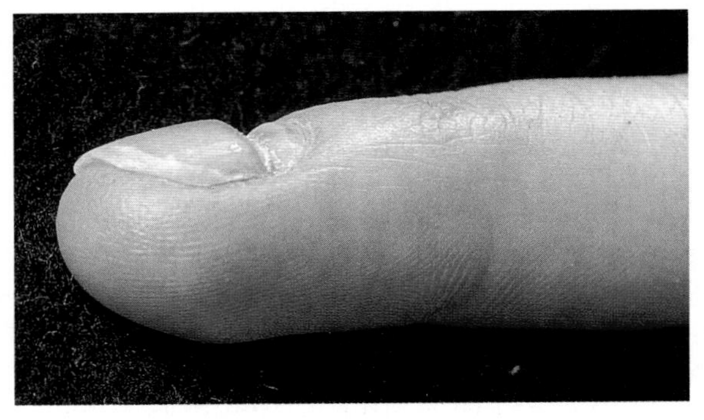

Fig. 7.7 Beau's lines—lateral view

disease. Beau's lines have been reported in severe zinc deficiency associated with acrodermatitis enteropathica (Weismann, 1977).

Onycholysis

This was originally associated with hyperthyroidism (Luria and Asper, 1958) and hypothyroidism (Fox, 1940), but may also be seen in Raynaud's disease, porphyria and yellow nail syndrome.

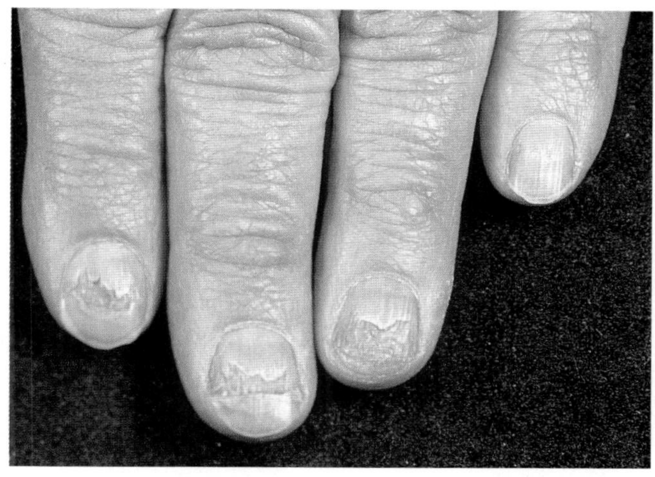

Fig. 7.8 Beau's lines—severe and leading to temporary loss of nail

Splinter haemorrhages

Although splinter haemorrhages have come to be associated with subacute bacterial endocarditis (Horder, 1920), they are by no means pathognomonic and are seen in many other conditions. They are commonly due to trauma (Gross and Tall, 1963) and are frequently seen in psoriasis, dermatitis and fungal infections of the nails. Splinter haemorrhages occur in many other medical conditions including trichinosis, rheumatoid arthritis, mitral stenosis, malignant neoplasms, severe anaemia, septicaemia (Fig. 7.9), dialysis and following renal transplantation.

Colour changes in general medicine

White

White nails have been described in hepatic cirrhosis (Terry, 1954a) (Fig. 7.10). The white colour is in the nail bed rather than the nail plate and is therefore quite different from leukonychia. The nails exhibit a ground glass-like opacity of most of the nail bed. The lunula is obscured, but there may be a

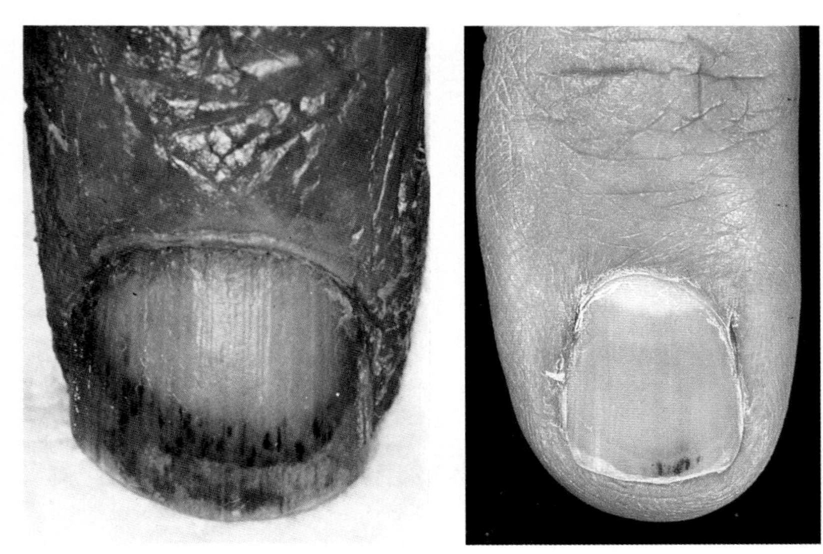

Fig. 7.9 Splinter haemorrhages in septicaemia

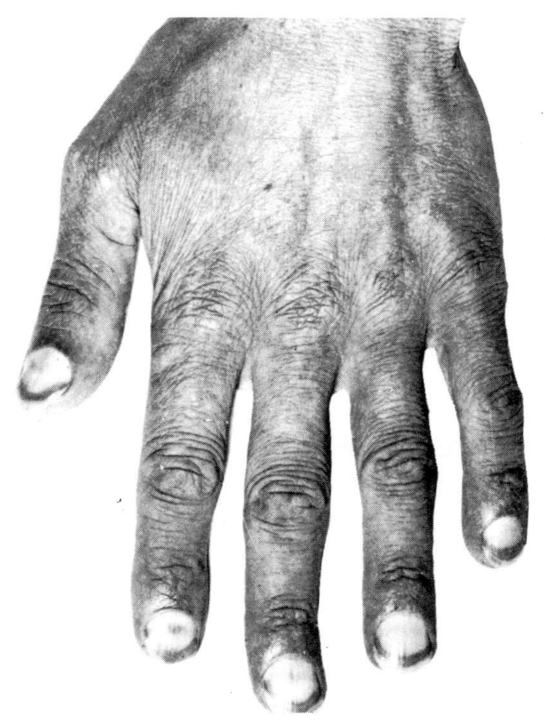

Fig. 7.10 White nails in patient convalescent from chronic hypoalbuminaemia (polycystic kidneys)

normal pink zone near the distal edge of the nail. The condition affects all nails symmetrically. Sometimes the white area may have a central peak distally (Morey and Burke, 1955). Flattening of the nail (platonychia) is also a frequent finding in hepatic cirrhosis. The nail beds may also be pale due to associated anaemia.

Paired white narrow bands may be seen in patients with chronic hypoalbuminaemia (Muehrcke, 1956). The bands run parallel with the lunula and are separated from one another and from the lunula by areas of normal pink nail. They do not move forward with the nail and therefore cannot be in the nail plate. The reason for their appearance is unknown and they are by no means always present in hypoalbuminaemia, but are most frequently seen in the nephrotic syndrome. They disappear if the serum albumin level is corrected and reappear on relapse.

Similar transverse white bands have been reported in zinc deficiency (the latter may be secondary to hypoalbuminaemia since zinc is largely protein bound) (Ferrandiz *et al.*, 1981). Juel-Jensen (1975) points out that persons suffering semi-starvation while on an expedition develop white bands on their nails corresponding in width to the period of deprivation. The condition is probably due to protein deficiency.

The 'half and half' nail seen in uraemia consists of a proximal dull white portion obliterating the lunula and a distal pink or brown portion with a well-demarcated transverse line of separation (Lindsay, 1967) (Fig. 7.11). Leyden and Wood (1972) showed that the pigment is melanin (and suggests that the cause is due to stimulation of melanocytes in the nail matrix by sudden renal decompensation). Only about 10% of chronic renal failure patients show this abnormality and it has no correlation with severity of uraemia (Daniel, Bower and Daniel, 1975). Similar changes have been described as brown nail bed arcs (Stewart and Raffle, 1972). There is no correlation between the size of nail bed arc and the serum creatinine level. The pigmentation does not grow out with the nail and would appear to be in the nail bed rather than nail plate.

Leukonychia affecting the nail plate has been seen in patients following treatment of renal failure (Hudson and Dennis, 1966) and associated with renal transplantation (Linder, 1978).

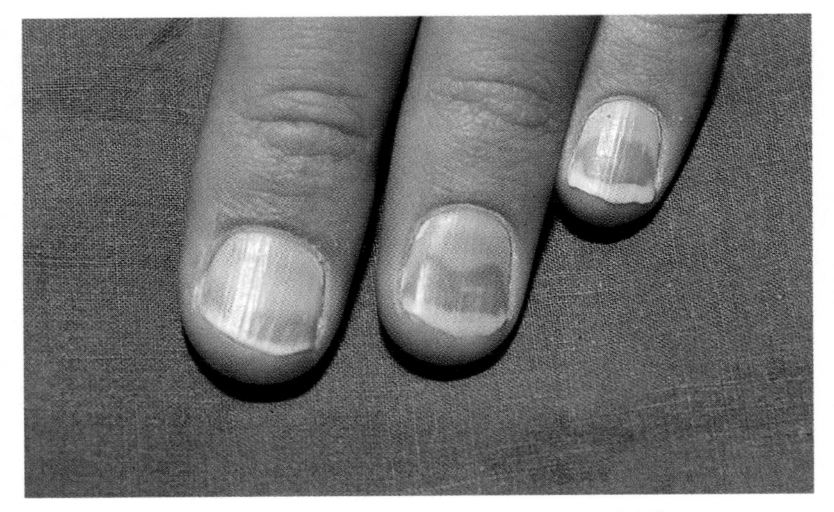

Fig. 7.11 'Half and half' nail in chronic renal failure

Colour changes in lunulae

Red or suffused halfmoons were described by Terry (1954b) in association with congestive cardiac failure. Similar changes are seen in alopecia areata.

Azure lunulae occur in Wilson's disease (hepatolenticular degeneration) (Bearn and McKusick, 1958) and are similar to those seen in argyria and phenolphthalein intake.

Pigmentation

Longitudinal bands of pigmentation affecting the nail beds associated with fingertip pigmentation are seen in Peutz-Jeghers syndrome (Valero and Sherf, 1965).

Digital and nail pigmentation may occur in vitamin B_{12} deficiency, but its correction produces resolution of the pigmentation.

Cutaneous hyperpigmentation is commonly seen in primary adrenal insufficiency, but occasionally nail pigmentation is also seen (Allenby and Snell, 1966). Longitudinal pigmentation of the nails has been reported following adrenalectomy for Cushing's syndrome (Bondy and Harwick, 1969).

Dark brown longitudinal bands in the nails have been described in India as a sign of malnutrition (Bisht and Singh, 1962); however, since pigmented bands are very common in dark-skinned persons their importance as a sign of malnutrition is probably small.

Well-water with a high elemental iron content may produce chromonychia; also the author has seen yellow staining of toe nails due to the high iron content of water in the River Irinoco (Olsen and Jattow, 1984).

Peripheral vascular disease

The nail is in a vulnerable site and is easily damaged by a reduced circulation. Cold-induced vascular spasm may produce several different changes in the nails. Arteriography has demonstrated that the same changes can be produced by both prolonged arterial spasm and digital artery occlusion (Samman and Strickland, 1962; Strickland and Urquhart, 1963).

Established Raynaud's disease of several years' duration will produce characteristic features. The nail plate becomes thin with longitudinal ridging which splits easily (Fig. 7.12).

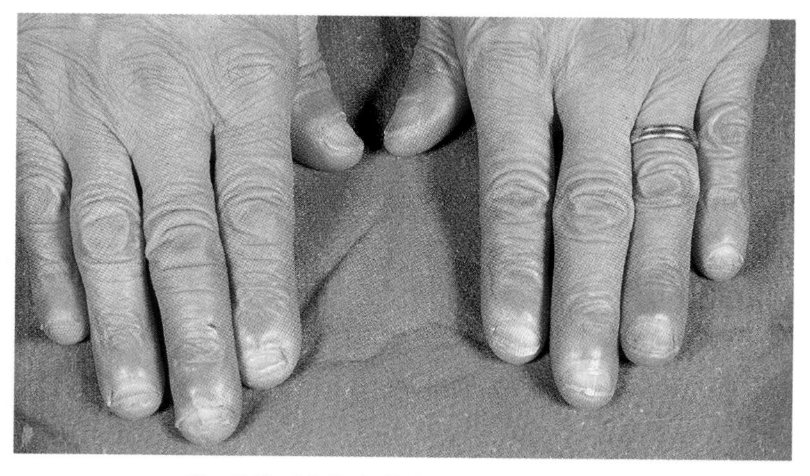

Fig. 7.12 Nails in Raynaud's syndrome

Koilonychia and onycholysis can occur and rarely thickening of the nail plate may develop, particularly in older patients. Secondary infection and accumulation of debris often produces discoloration. Nail growth may be slightly decreased.

Excessive exposure to cold in patients with Raynaud's disease can produce Beau's lines due to a temporary cessation of nail growth, but not all nails are affected (unlike Beau's lines seen in general medical disorders, see p. 115). Partial or total

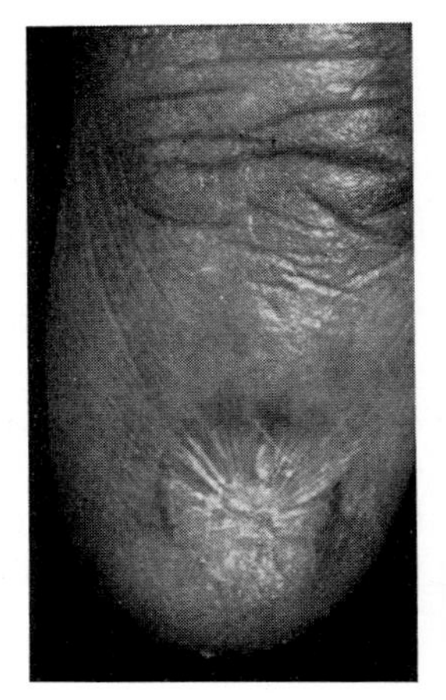

Fig. 7.13 Permanent loss of nail due to digital artery occlusion

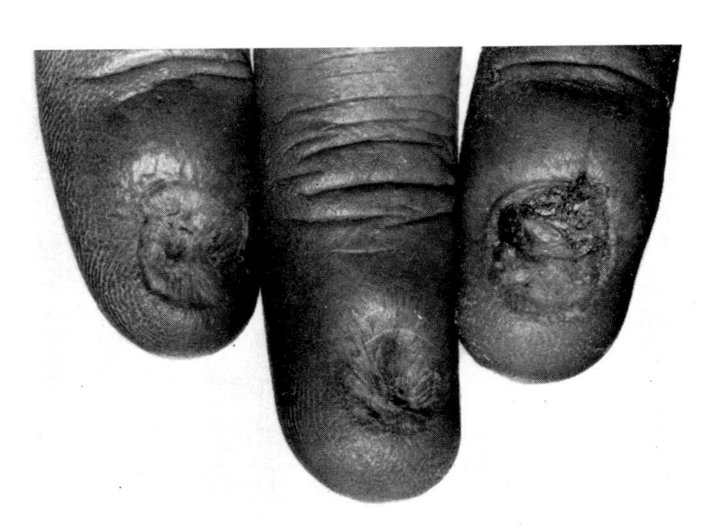

Fig. 7.14 Permanent loss of several nails associated with severe Raynaud's symptoms but no arterial occlusion

loss of the nails may be seen in diabetes and scleroderma. Permanent shedding of the nail plate with scarring affecting a single digit can occur as a result of digital artery occlusion (Fig. 7.13), or affecting several digits in generalised severe spasm (Fig. 7.14). A less common change, pterygium formation, is seen particularly in vasomotor ischaemia (Edwards, 1948) (Fig. 7.15), although other causes such as lichen planus must be excluded.

Patients with cold hands often have chronic paronychia and *Candida albicans* may complicate the picture with involvement of the nail plate.

The treatment of these disorders is the treatment of the underlying condition. Inositol nicotinate 250 mg three or four times daily has been of value in some cases. Improvement may only be slight and other vasodilators may be tried. Recent studies have claimed success with use of topical glyceryl trinitrate (Percutol) and nifedipine (Pierce, Valle and Wielenga, 1983). Holti has successfully used ultraviolet light, producing a brisk erythema in 8–24 hours on each exposure. The treatment needs to be given annually at the onset of cold weather.

For organic arterial occlusion, infusions of low molecular weight dextran or heparin may be useful (Holti, 1965).

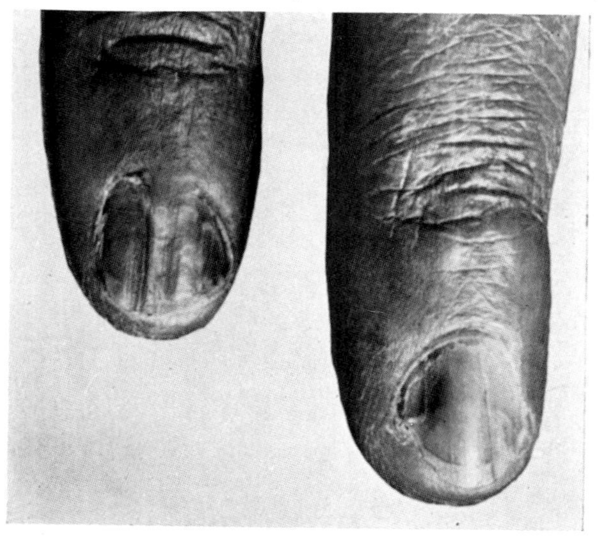

Fig. 7.15 Raynaud's symptoms—early pterygium formation

Connective tissue disease

Ridging and beading (Fig. 7.16) has been shown to occur more often in patients with rheumatoid arthritis (especially over 30 years of age) than in normal subjects (Hamilton, 1960). The fact that it occurs in quite a high proportion of normal people and is much commoner in old age than in youth, makes it doubtful if its occurrence in rheumatoid arthritis is of any great significance. Rheumatoid vasculitis results in small infarcts around the nails, nail folds and fingertips (Bywaters and Scott 1963). Splinter haemorrhages are common in the nail folds. Areas of periungual ischaemia may resemble superficial paronychia (O'Quinn, Kennedy and Baker, 1965). Yellow nail syndrome has been described in association with rheumatoid arthritis.

Nail fold telangiectasia and erythema with hyperkeratotic irregular cuticles are characteristic of dermatomyositis (Samitz, 1974) (Figs. 7.17, 7.18, 7.19).

Clubbing, splinter haemorrhages, nail fold infarcts, onycholysis and nail plate changes such as pitting, ridging and leukonychia can occur in lupus erythematosus (Mackie, 1973; Urowitz *et al.*, 1978).

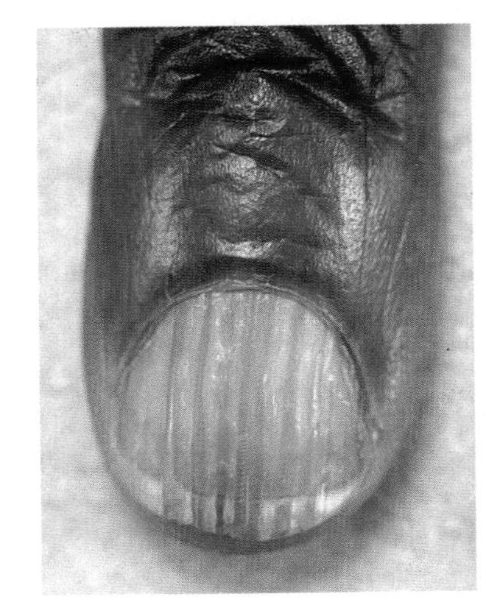

Fig. 7.16 Ridging and beading

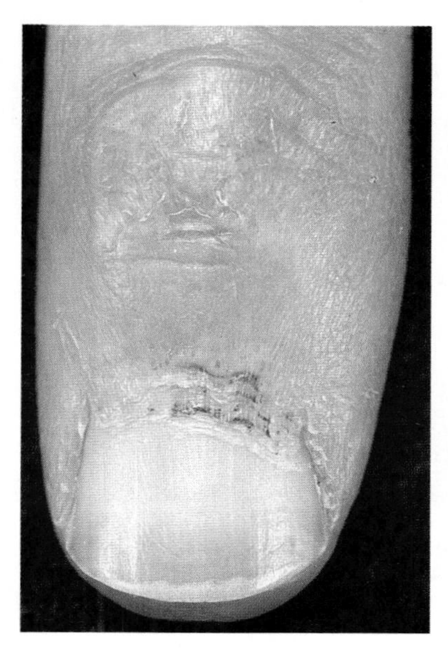

Fig. 7.17 Dermatomyositis—nail fold changes

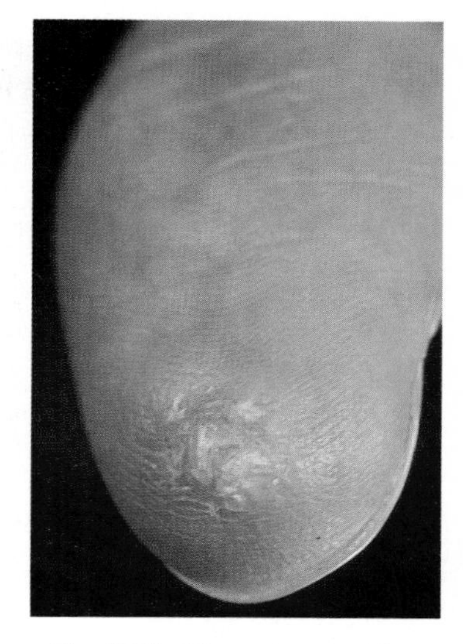

Fig. 7.18 Dermatomyositis—calcinosis

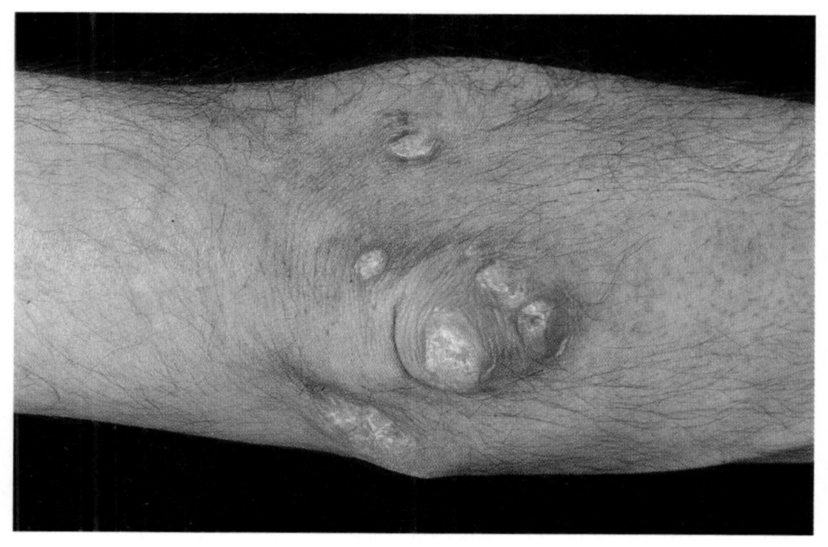

Fig. 7.19 Dermatomyositis—calcinosis

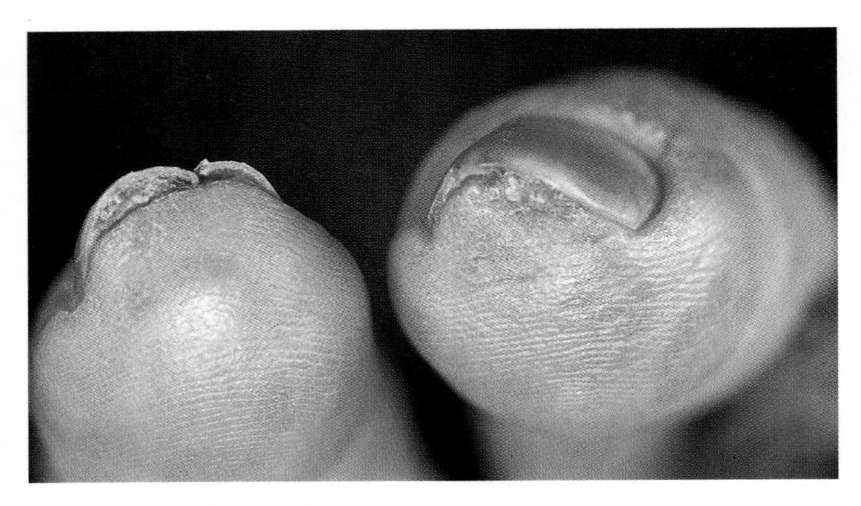

Fig. 7.20 Pterygium inversum ungius in SLE

Nail fold telangiectasia, erythema and digital infarcts may occur in scleroderma. Pterygium inversum unguis is seen in scleroderma and SLE (Fig. 7.20).

The yellow nail syndrome

This is the name given by Samman and White (1964) to a rather characteristic condition. Patients notice that their nails cease, or almost cease, to grow and some months later take on a yellow or greenish colour. Although the colour usually affects the whole nail plate, occasionally the proximal part of the nail may be of normal hue. The changes affect both finger nails and toe nails. The nails normally remain smooth and may be somewhat thickened. They may be excessively curved from side to side, the lateral margins are less covered by soft tissue than in normal nails, and the cuticle is usually deficient (Fig. 7.21). One or more nails may show a distinctive hump (Fig. 7.22). Onycholysis often affects one or more nails and may extend so far towards the matrix that the nail plate is shed. It is very slowly replaced. In a few cases there are ridges across the nails indicating variations in their rate of growth but overall the rate of growth is very slow, being reduced to

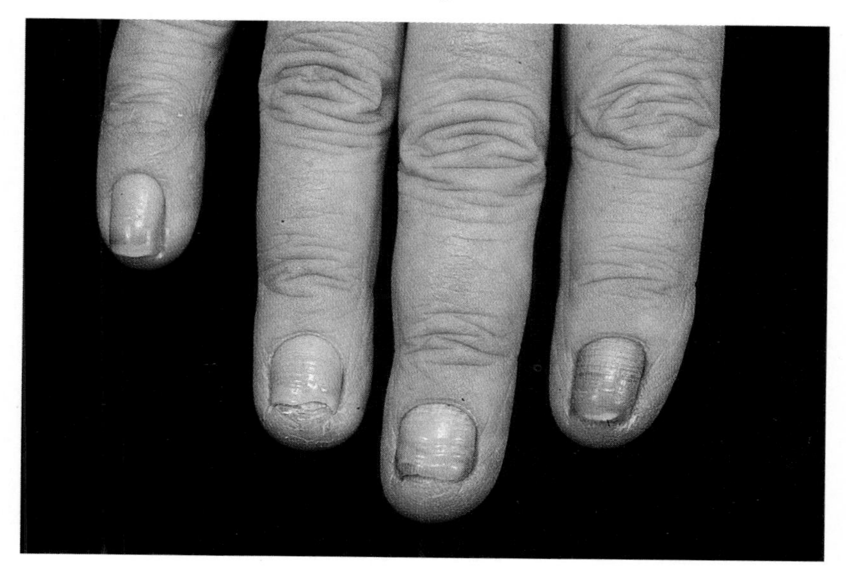

Fig. 7.21 Nails in yellow nail syndrome

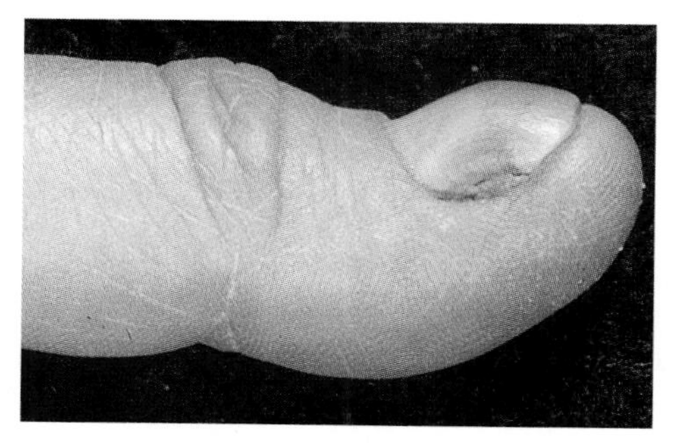

Fig. 7.22 'Hump' in yellow nail syndrome

0.25 mm per week or less (compared with 0.5 mm, lower limit of normal).

In addition to the changes in the nails themselves, there is usually some oedema. This may be confined to the fingertips but is often more widespread. The ankles are often swollen and there may be facial oedema. Occasionally very severe oedema is seen. Lymphangiography may show atresia of lymphatic vessels or a single varicose vessel as seen in primary lymphoedema. However, in some patients, even with severe oedema clinically, the vessels appear normal on lymphangiography.

Many patients also have some chest symptoms. Chronic bronchitis is most common, but bronchiectasis is not infrequent (Dilley *et al.*, 1968) and pleural effusions are occasionally found (Emerson, 1966). Sinusitis may also occur. It has also been suggested that patients with the yellow nail syndrome are liable to develop malignant neoplasms. Reported associated malignancies have included melanoma, Hodgkin's disease, sarcoma, and laryngeal and endometrial carcinoma. Immunological abnormalities such as hypogammaglobulinaemia may rarely be encountered.

Treatment of this disorder is unrewarding. Supportive treatment may improve the appearance of the proximal part of the nails while the distal portion remains discoloured. Complete spontaneous recovery in the appearance of the nails has occasionally been seen. Partial or complete recovery occurs in 30% of patients but there may be a relapse. The improved appearance of the nails is accompanied by a return to normal rate of growth of the nails. Vitamin E may sometimes produce resolution (Fig. 7.23).

Shell nail syndrome

Cornelius and Shelley (1967) describe a patient who developed bronchiectasis at the age of 4 years following whooping cough, and at the age of 5 finger nail changes were noted, all showing longitudinal curvature of nail plate with onycholysis. There was also atrophy of the distal nail bed. There seems to be little difference between this condition and some cases of yellow nail syndrome.

HIV Infection

Various changes in the nail plate have been reported in patients with AIDS, including varying degrees of hyperpigmentation, transverse and longitudinal ridging, changes in size of lunula, and onycholysis. Yellowing of the nails was seen in four of eight patients with AIDS and *Pneumocystis carinii* pneumonia (Chernosky and Finlay, 1985) although it is unlikely that this represents true yellow nail syndrome (Scher, 1988).

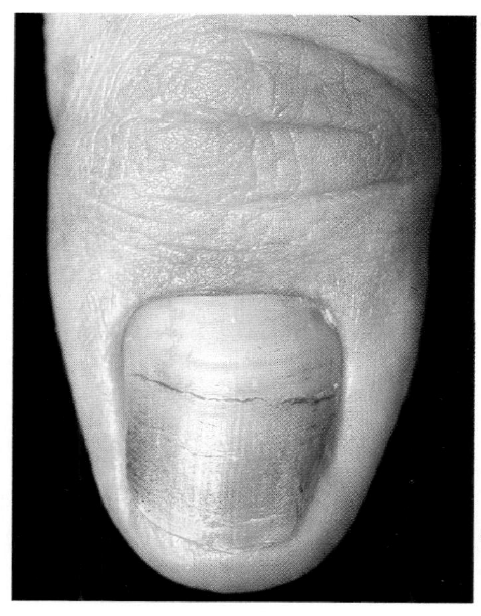

Fig. 7.23(a) and (b) Yellow nail syndrome—spontaneous resolution with normal regrowth

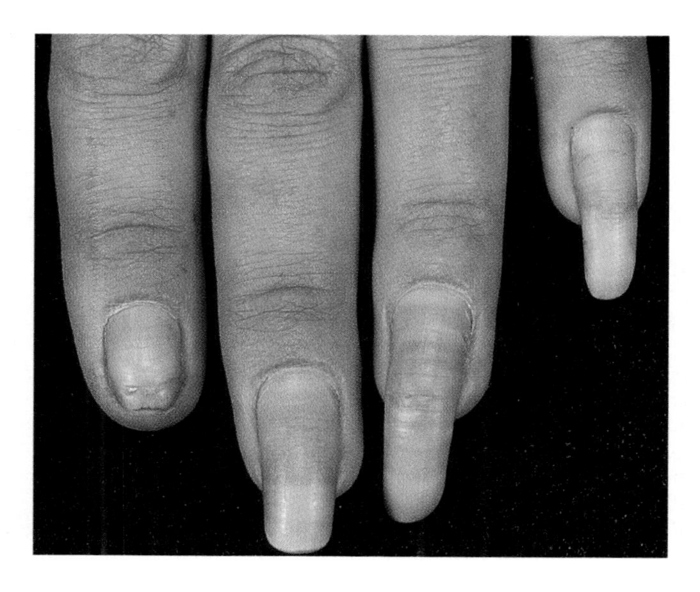

References

Allenby, C P and Snell, P H (1966) Longitudinal pigmentation of the nails in Addison's Disease. *Brit. Med. J.* **1** 1582

Bearn, A G and McKusick, V A (1958) Azure lunulae. *J. Amer. Med. Assoc.* **166** 904

Beau, J H S (1846) Certain caracteres de semeliologie retrospective, presentes par les ongles. *Arch. Gen. Med.* **9** 447

Bentley-Phillips, B and Bayles, M A H (1971) Occupational koilonychia of the toe nails. *Brit. J. Derm.* **85** 149

Beutler, E (1964) Tissue effects of iron deficiency. In *Iron Metabolism* (ed Gross, F). Berlin, Gottingen, Heidelberg: Springer-Verlag

Bisht, D B and Singh, S S (1962) Pigmented bands on nails. A new sign of malnutrition. *Lancet* **i** 507

Bondy, P K and Harwick, H J (1969) Longitudinal banded pigmentation of nails following adrenalectomy for Cushing's syndrome. *New Eng. J. Med.* **281** 1056

Bywaters, E G L and Scott, J T (1963) The Natural History of vascular lesions in rheumatoid arthritis. *J. Chron. Disease* **16** 905–914

Chernosky, M E and Finlay, V K (1985) Yellow nail syndrome in patients with acquired immunodeficiency disease. *J. Amer. Acad. Derm.* **13** 731–736

Comaish, J S (1965) Diseases of nails. *Newcastle Med. J.* **28** 253

Cornelius, C E III and Shelley, W B (1967) Shell nail syndrome associated with bronchiectasis. *Arch. Derm.* **96** 694

Daniel, C R, Bower, J D and Daniel, C R Jr (1975) The half and half fingernail. A clue to chronic renal failure. *Mississippi State Med. Assoc.* **16** 367

Dawber, R (1974) Occupational koilonychia. *Brit. J. Derm.* **91 Suppl. 10** 11

Dilley, J J, Kierland, R R, Randall, R V and Shick, A M (1968) Primary lymphedema associated with yellow nails and pleural effusion. *J. Am. Med. Assoc.* **204** 122

Edwards, E A (1948) Nail changes in functional and organic arterial disease. *New Eng. J. Med.* **239** 362

Emerson, P A (1966) Yellow nails, lymphoedema and pleural effusions. *Thorax* **21** 247

Ferrandiz, C, Hennes, J, Peyri, J and Sarmiento, J (1981) Acquired zinc deficiency syndrome during total parenteral alimentation. *Derm.* **163** 255

Fox, E C (1940) Disease of the nails. Report of cases of onycholysis. *Arch. Derm.* **41** 98

Gross, N J and Tall, R (1963) Clinical significance of splinter haemorrhages. *Brit. Med. J.* **2** 1496

Hall, G H (1959) The cause of digital clubbing. Testing a new hypothesis. *Lancet* **i** 750

Hamilton, E D B (1960) Nail studies in rheumatoid arthritis. *Ann. Rheum. Dis.* **19** 167

Handa, Y, Handa, K, Koaka, S and Mitani, S (1960) A note in the genetics of koilonychia. *Acta Genet. Med. Gemell.* **9** 309

Hellier, F F (1950) Hereditary koilonychia. *Brit. J. Derm.* **62** 213

Holti, G (1965) The effect of intermittent low molecular dextran upon the digital circulation in systemic sclerosis. *Brit. J. Derm.* **77** 560

Horder, T (1920) Discussion on clinical significance and course of subacute bacterial endocarditis. *Brit. Med. J.* **2** 301

Hudson, J B and Dennis, A J (1966) Transverse white lines in the fingernails after acute and chronic renal failure. *Arch. Intern. Med.* **117** 276

Jalili, M A and Al-Kassab, S (1959) Koilonychia and cystine content of nails. *Lancet* **ii** 108

Juel-Jensen, B E (1975) Expedition nails. *Brit. Med. J.* **2** 140

Leyden, J J and Wood, M G (1972) The half and half nail of uraemic onychodystrophy. *Arch. Derm.* **105** 591

Linder, M (1978) Striped nails after kidney transplant. *Ann. Intern. Med.* **88** 809

Lindsay, P G (1967) The half-and-half nail. *Arch. Intern. Med.* **119** 583

Luria, M N and Asper, S P Jr (1958) Onycholysis in hyperthyroidism. *Ann. Intern. Med.* **49** 102

Mackie, R M (1973) Lupus erythematosus in association with finger clubbing. *Brit. J. Derm.* **89** 533

Morey, D A J and Burke, J O (1955) Distinctive nail changes in advanced hepatic cirrhosis. *Gastroenterol.* **29** 258

Muehrcke, R C (1956) The finger nails in chronic hypoalbuminaemia. *Brit. Med. J.* **1** 1327

O'Quinn, S E, Kennedy, C B and Baker, D T (1965) Peripheral vascular lesions in rheumatoid arthritis. *Arch. Derm.* **92** 489

Olsen, T G and Jattow, P (1984) Contact exposure to elemental iron causing chromonychia. *Arch. Derm.* **120** 120

Pierce, E H, Valle, R D and Wielenga, J (1983) Raynaud's disease and nifedipine. *Ann. Intern. Med.* **97** 111

Samitz, M H (1974) Cuticular changes in dermatomyositis. *Arch. Derm.* **110** 866

Samman, P D and Strickland, B (1962) Abnormalities of the fingernails associated with impaired peripheral blood supply. *Brit. J. Derm.* **74** 163

Samman, P D and White, W F (1964) The yellow nail syndrome. *Brit. J. Derm.* **76** 53

Scher, R K (1988) Acquired immunodeficiency syndrome and yellow nails. *J. Amer. Acad. Derm.* **18** 758–759

Stewart, W K and Raffle, E J (1972) Brown nail-bed arcs and chronic renal disease. *Brit. Med. J.* **1** 784

Strickland, B and Urquhart, W (1963) Digital arteriography with reference to nail dystrophy. *Brit. J. Radiol.* **36** 465

Stone, O J (1975) Spoon nails and clubbing. Significance and mechanisms. *Cutis.* **16** 235

Stone, O J and Maberry, J D (1965) Spoon nails and clubbing. Review and possible mechanisms. *Texas State J. Med.* **61** 620

Terry, R (1954a) White nails in hepatic cirrhosis. *Lancet* **i** 757

Terry, R (1954b) Red half-moons in cardiac failure. *Lancet* **ii** 842

Urowitz, M B, Gladman, D D, Chalmers, A and Ogryzlo, M A (1978) Nail lesions in systemic lupus erythematosus. *J. Rheumatol.* **5** 441

Valero, A and Sherf, K (1965) Pigmented nails in Peutz-Jeghers syndrome. *Amer. J. Gastroenterol.* **43** 56

Weismann, K (1977) Lines of Beau—possible marker of zinc deficiency. *Acta. Derm. Venereol. (Stock.)* **59** 88

Young, J R (1966) Ulcerative colitis and finger-clubbing. *Brit. Med. J.* **1** 278

8

Nail changes due to drugs

D. A. Fenton

Antimalarial agents

In addition to cutaneous pigmentation, discoloration of the nails is seen with chloroquine therapy. The colour varies from blue-grey to yellow. The nails also fluoresce under Wood's light, even in the absence of obvious pigmentation in daylight. Mepacrine produces similar changes.

Discoloration is seen more easily in Caucasians and may still be present for many months after discontinuing the drug (Tuffanelli, Abraham and Dubois, 1963).

Antibiotics

Photosensitivity, painful photo-onycholysis and yellow pigmentation affecting several nails have been reported with dimethylchlortetracycline and doxycycline, and rarely with chlortetracycline and oxytetracycline (Segal, 1963). Strong sunlight is required to induce the change which is often accompanied by considerable discomfort. Yellow fluorescence of nails under Wood's light can be seen with prolonged tetracycline therapy. Minocycline causes cutaneous pigmentation and blue-grey pigmentation of the nail bed.

Temporary loss has been described as due to large doses of cloxacillin and cephaloridine (Eastwood *et al.*, 1969).

Onycholysis has been reported in association with chloramphenicol therapy (Norton, 1980; Runne and Orfanos, 1981).

Oral contraceptives

The oral contraceptive pill may cause photo-onycholysis in patients with porphyria cutanea tarda or porphyria variegata. Occasionally an increase in nail growth rate and less splitting and chipping occurs in some women taking the oral contraceptive pill.

Phenothiazines

High doses of chlorpromazine produce blue-black or purple pigmentation of the nail beds in addition to pigmentation of exposed areas of skin. This may be more obvious in the summer months (Stanlove, 1965).

Beta-blockers

Practolol has been shown to be responsible for a psoriasiform nail dystrophy associated with onycholysis and subungual hyperkeratosis. Ventral pterygium formation and over-curvature of the nails has also been described (Tegner, 1976).

Propranolol has also produced psoriasiform eruptions associated with thickening, pitting and discoloration of the nails. Metoprolol has been associated with the occurrence of alopecia and Beau's lines.

Timolol maleate eyedrops sometimes cause nail pigmentation associated with discoloration of the digits (Feiler-Offry, Godel and Lazar, 1981).

Psoralens

Longitudinal and diffuse pigmentation of the nails may occur with systemic 8-methoxypsoralen therapy. Photo-onycholysis with subungual haemorrhage may also be seen (Naik and Singh, 1979; Zala, Omar and Krebs, 1977) (Fig. 8.1).

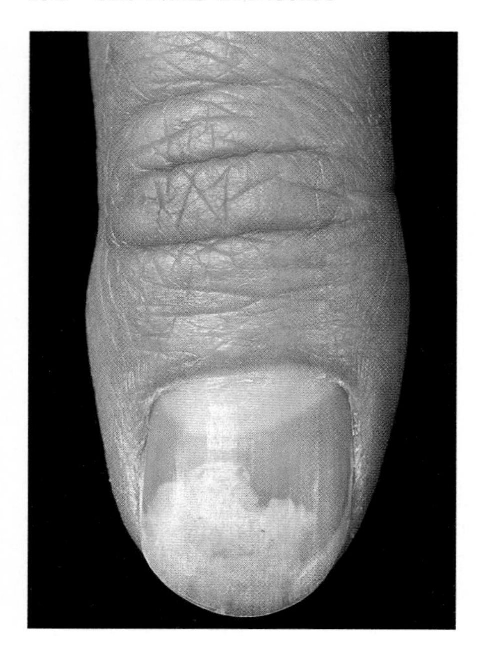

Fig. 8.1 Photo-onycholysis

Retinoids

Paronychia and increased nail fragility have been recognised as side-effects of aromatic retinoid therapy (Baran, Brun and Juhlin, 1983). Nail growth rate may also be affected and Beau's lines can also occur (Ferguson, Simpson and Hammersley, 1983). Excessive granulation tissue and ingrowing toe nails have been associated with retinoid therapy (Campbell *et al.*, 1983).

Arsenic

Transverse broad white lines (Mees' lines) may be seen after acute arsenic poisoning. Single or multiple lines can occur. Analysis of the lines for arsenic is used to date the time of exposure to the poison (Pounds, Pearson and Turner, 1979).

Phenolphthalein

The fixed drug eruption of phenolphthalein will produce a dark blue colour if it occurs on the nail bed. (Wise and Sulzberger, 1933). Phenolphthalein used in purgatives can cause azure lunulae (as seen in argyria) (Campbell, 1931). Purgative abuse has produced reversible finger clubbing (Levine, Wingate and Goode, 1981).

Argyria

Systemic argyrosis produces blue discoloration of the lunulae (identical with that seen in Wilson's disease) associated with blue-grey cutaneous pigmentation (Ronchese, 1959).

Gold

Gold can cause thin, brittle nails with longitudinal streaking and yellow-brown discoloration (Fam and Paton, 1984). Onycholysis may also occur.

Benoxaprofen

Benoxaprofen produced photosensitivity associated with reversible onycholysis. Increased nail growth and hypertrichosis are also seen in some patients (Fenton, English and Wilkinson, 1982).

D-Penicillamine

Yellow nail syndrome has been reported in association with D-penicillamine therapy (Ilchyshyn and Vickers, 1983).

Cytotoxics

Cytotoxic therapy produces a variety of nail changes. Diffuse, transverse or longitudinal pigmentation of nail can occur with most cytotoxic agents. There may be associated cutaneous pigmentation and alopecia, and splinter haemorrhages and Beau's lines are also seen. Diffuse and transverse leukonychia have been described, although this appears to be less common. Blue discoloration is often seen in HIV patients treated with AZT. Onycholysis and shedding of nails may also occur (Scher and Daniel, 1990).

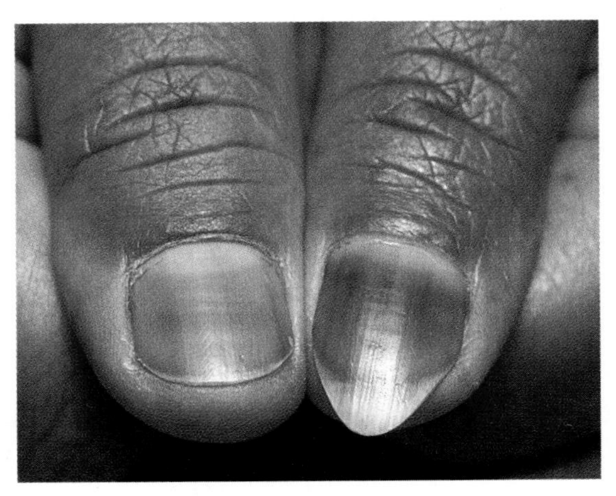

Fig. 8.2 Chromonychia while on Tamoxifen

Lithium carbonate

Colour changes and 'dystrophic' alterations have been reported with lithium therapy (Don and Silverman, 1988).

References

Baran, R, Brun, P and Juhlin, L (1983) Leuconychie transversale induite par étrétinale. *Ann. Derm.* **109** 367

Campbell, G (1931) Peculiar pigmentation following use of a purgative containing phenolphthalein. *Brit. J. Derm.* **43** 186

Campbell, J P, Grekin, R C, Ellis, C N *et al.* (1983) Retinoid therapy is associated with excess granulation tissue responses. *J. Amer. Acad. Derm.* **9** 708

Don, P C and Silverman, R A (1988) Nail dystrophy caused by lithium carbonate. *Cutis* **41** 19

Eastwood, J B, Curtis, J R, Smith, E K M and Wardener, H E De (1969) Shedding of nails apparently induced by administration of large amounts of cephaloridine and cloxacillin in two anephric patients. *Brit. J. Derm.* **81** 750

Fam, A G and Paton, T W (1984) Nail pigmentation after parenteral gold therapy for rheumatoid arthritis: gold nails. *Arth. Rheum.* **27** 119

Feiler-Offry, V, Godel, V and Lazar, M (1981) Nail pigmentation following timolol maleate therapy. *Ophthalmologica, Basle* **182** 153

Fenton, D A, English, J S and Wilkinson, J D (1982) Hypertrichosis and increased nail and hair growth following treatment with benoxaprofen. *Brit. Med. J.* **284** 1228

Ferguson, M M, Simpson, N B and Hammersley, N (1983) Severe nail dystrophy associated with retinoid therapy. *Lancet* **ii** 974

Ilchyshyn, A and Vickers, C F H (1983) Yellow nail syndrome associated with penicillamine therapy. *Acta Derm. Venereol. (Stock.)* **63** 554

Levine, D, Wingate, D L and Goode, A W (1981) Purgative abuse associated with reversible cachexia, hypogammaglobulinaemia and finger clubbing. *Lancet* **i** 919

Naik, R P C and Singh, G (1979) Nail pigmentation due to oral 8-methoxypsoralen. *Brit. J. Derm.* **100** 229

Norton, L A (1980) Nail disorders. *J. Amer. Acad. Derm.* **2** 451

Pounds, C A, Pearson, F F and Turner, T D (1979) Arsenic in fingernails. *J. Forens. Sci. Soc.* **19** 165

Ronchese, F (1959) Argyrosis and cyanosis-melanosis and cyanosis. *Arch. Derm.* **80** 227

Runne, U and Orfanos, C (1981) The human nail. *Curr. Prob. Derm.* **9** 102

Scher, R K and Daniel, C R (1990) *Nails: Therapy, Diagnosis, Surgery*. London: Saunders

Segal, B M (1963) Photosensitivity, nail discoloration and onycholysis. *Arch. Int. Med.* **112** 165

Stanlove, A (1965) Pigmentation due to phenothiazines in high and prolonged dosage. *J. Amer. Med. Assoc.* **191** 263

Tegner, E (1976) Reversible overcurvature of nails after treatment with practolol. *Acta Derm. Venereol. (Stock.)* **56** 493

Tuffanelli, D, Abraham, R K and Dubois, E I (1963) Pigmentation from antimalarial therapy. *Arch. Derm.* **88** 113

Wise, F and Sulzberger, M B (1933) Drug eruptions: fixed phenolphthalein eruptions. *Arch. Derm.* **27** 549

Zala, L, Omar, A and Krebs, A (1977) Photo-onycholysis induced by 8-methoxypsoralen. *Dermatologica* **154** 203

9

The nail and cosmetics

R. Baran and R. P. R. Dawber

The application of nail cosmetics may cause injury to the nail and surrounding tissues and reactions at distant sites. In this chapter the basic ingredients of nail preparations are considered together with the pathological changes sometimes induced by them. In assessing eczematous and other periungual reactions it is important also to realise that nail tissues, particularly the subungual and paronychial areas, may be 'reservoirs' for small amounts of cosmetic preparations applied by hand to other parts of the skin; these may cause nail apparatus abnormalities.

Nail polish

The term nail lacquer is sometimes used to include enamels, top coats, and base coats, either as separate entities or combined in one product. The base coat is a material used to improve the adhesion or bonding of enamel to the nail. A top coat improves the depth and lustre of the enamel and increases its resistance to chipping and abrasion. Nail polishes consist of solids and solvent ingredients, the former representing about 30%, the latter 70% of the product. Essentially, the ingredients can be divided into six principal groups:

(1) Cellulose film formers, such as nitrocellulose. These give gloss, body and gel structure.

(2) Resins to improve the gloss and adhesion of the film, such as toluene sulphonamide-formaldehyde resin.

(3) Plasticisers added to give the film pliability, to minimise shrinkage, and soften and plasticise the cellulose, such as dibutylphthalate.

(4) Thixotropic suspending agents for non-settling and flow, such as bentonite; they keep pigments in suspension on shaking.

(5) Solvents (such as butyl acetate) and diluents (such as toluene) which keep nitrocellulose, resin, and plasticiser in a liquid state and control the application and drying time.

(6) Colouring substances. These are either inorganic (iron oxides) or a variety of certified organic colours (D and C yellow Al lakes). In principle they require to be insoluble in a nail lacquer system.

'Pearls' or 'frosts' are produced by bismuth oxychloride and titanium dioxide coated with mica and guanine, obtained from fish scales. 'Clears' contain a small tint.

The base coat is formulated in a manner similar to standard lacquer but it has a lower non-volatile content (less nitrocellulose) and a lower viscosity since a thinner film is desirable; it may also contain hydrolysed gelatin.

In the top coat the nitrocellulose content is increased, and the resin is reduced. A slight increase in plasticiser content improves elasticity of the film. There is no pigment. The top coat often has an added sunscreen.

Reactions

Nail varnish dermatitis

Frequently nail polish dermatitis of allergic origin appears on any part of the body accessible to the nails, with no signs in or around the nail apparatus. The commonest areas involved are the eyelids, the lower half of the face, the sides of the neck, and the upper chest. Generalised dermatitis may rarely occur. Sometimes the use of nail polish on stockings to stop 'runs' or on nickel-plated costume jewellery to prevent nickel dermatitis may induce nail polish dermatitis respectively on the legs or at the site of the metal contact. Nail polish dermatitis may occur in the user's spouse or other close contacts.

Although any ingredient may account for distant allergic eczematous contact dermatitis, the thermoplastic resin is the most common culprit. After the nail polish is removed, the dermatitis usually clears rapidly unless secondary infection or lichenification has occurred.

Metal pellets put in some bottles to maintain a liquid state may cause nickel reactions and onycholysis.

Nail plate staining

Nail plate staining from the use of polish is most commonly yellow-orange in colour. It typically starts near the cuticle, extends to the nail tip and becomes progressively darker from base to tip. With the leaking out of the varnish, the dyes penetrate the nail too deeply to be removed.

Nail keratin granulation

Injury to the nail plate from nail lacquers is rare. However, 'granulation' of nail keratin, a superficial friability, can be observed in some instances where individuals leave nail lacquer on for many weeks, or due to poor formulation of the product.

Nail varnish patch testing

Several nail lacquers should be used and tested 'as is'; they should be allowed to dry for 15 minutes since the solvents and diluents may cause false positive reactions. The following substances should be included in the test battery:

aryl-sulphonamide formaldehyde resin (10% petrolatum)
nickel (0.5% petrolatum) DMG spot test for nickel
glyceryl phthalate resin (polymer resin) 10% petrolatum
pearly material–guanine powder (pure)
formaldehyde (1–2% in aqua)
colophony (resin) 10% petrolatum (Fisher) 20% (Cronin)
drometrizole (Tunuvin P) 1% petrolatum to 5%

The resin contains no free formaldehyde. Formaldehyde is merely the chemical moiety on which the resin is formed. Usually formaldehyde-sensitive individuals do not cross-react with this resin. However Dutch workers have suggested that there is always a small amount of free formaldehyde present in many preparations (Nater, de Groot, Liem, 1985). Various cosmetic companies make varnishes which are formulated without the sensitising resin, using alkyl resin as a substitute; unfortunately this tends to peel and chip.

Nail polish removers

These are composed of various solvents such as acetone. Occasionally nail polish removers cause trouble by excessive drying of the nail plate and may be responsible for some of the inflammations of paronychial skin.

Sculptured artificial nails (fingernail elongators)

Sculptured artificial nails are available in a set containing a template, a liquid monomer, and a powdered polymer. Self-curing acrylic resins are created by polymerisation of methyl methacrylate monomer and polymethyl methacrylate powder with an organic peroxide and an accelerator. They harden at room temperature. The compound has to be moulded on the natural nail. After it is roughened with a burr, the natural nail is painted with an acrylic compound, which when hardened produces a prosthetic nail that is enlarged and elongated by repeated applications. The prosthesis can be filed and manicured to shape, and as the nail plate grows out, further applications of acrylic can be made to maintain a regular contour.

Allergic contact dermatitis (Fig. 9.1) may occur, typically 2–4 months after the first application. The reaction may involve the face, eyelids, and dorsal aspect of some of the involved fingers as well as paronychial tissues. All cases complain of severe onychial and paronychial pain (Baran and Schibli, 1990; Fisher and Baran, 1991), sometimes associated with persistent paraesthesia, and, uncommonly, nail discoloration is seen. The

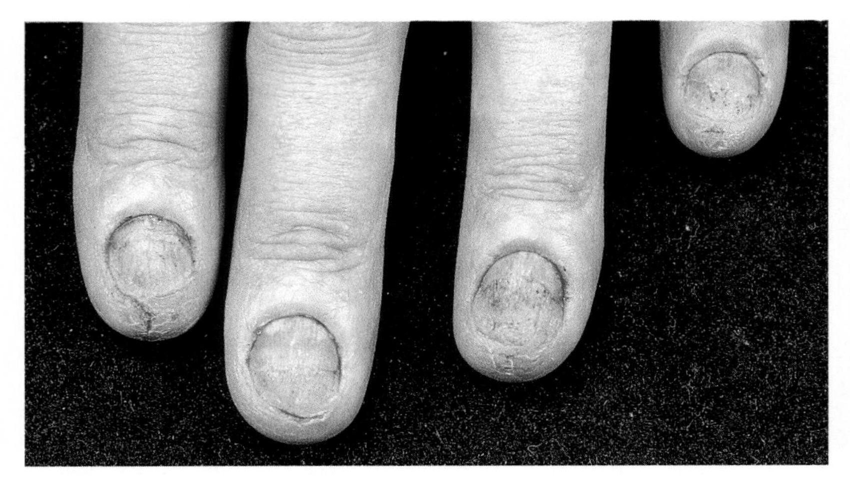

Fig. 9.1 Allergic contact dermatitis nail changes to acrylic resin artificial nails

nail bed can be dry and thickened. The nail dystrophy consists of onycholysis with thinning and splitting of the true nail. It may be several months before the nails return to normal.

Sculptured artificial nail patch testing shows allergic patients react strongly to the acrylic liquid monomer and not to the polymer—this is similar to denture allergy. Suggested allergens for testing should include:

methyl methacrylate monomer (10% in olive oil)
methacrylate acid esters (1% and 5% in olive oil and petrolatum)

Since acrylic monomers may cross-react, the newer products seem just as likely to cause allergic dermatitis.

Preformed plastic nails

Preformed plastic nails are packaged in several shapes and sizes to conform to the normal nail plate configuration. Such nails are trimmed to fit the fingertip and are fixed with a special adhesive supplied with the kit.

The usefulness of these prosthetic nails is limited by the need for some normal nail to be present for attachment.

Normal physical and chemical insults to the nails cause the preformed plastic nails to loosen unless the ethyl 2-cyanoacrylate adhesive is used. If the preformed nails remain in place for 3 or 4 days they may cause onycholysis, and nail surface damage (Fig. 9.2); less commonly, complete disruption of the nail may occur if the nail is left *in situ* for 3 or more days. The changes may be indistinguishable from those caused by formaldehyde nail hardeners. In some cases, distant allergic eczematous contact dermatitis of the face and eyelids has occurred.

On patch testing, the patients react far more often to the adhesive than to the prosthetic nails. Suggested test substances are:

paratertiary butyl phenol resin (1% petrolatum)
tricresyl ethyl phthalate (5% petrolatum)
cyanoacrylates
other glues (5% methyl ethyl ketone)

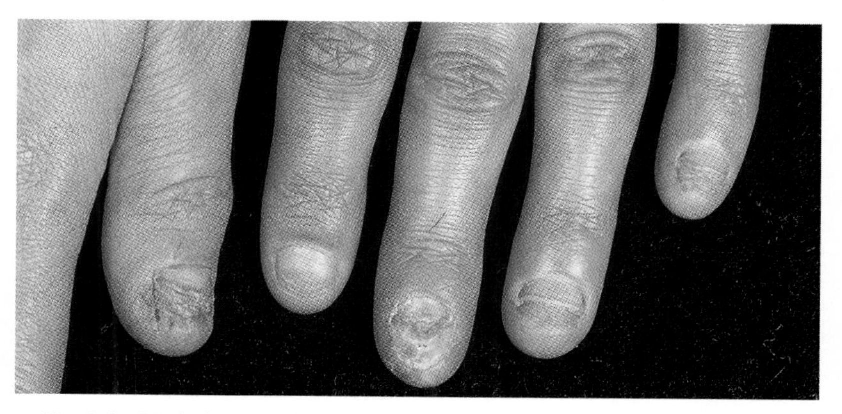

Fig. 9.2 Nail changes following application of adhesive for false nails

Nail hardeners

Nail keratin can be hardened by some tissue fixatives such as formaldehyde preparations. These are not commercially available in the United States because of their toxic effects.

Nail changes caused by such nail hardeners may include subungual haemorrhage and bluish discoloration of the nail.

The nail returns to normal when the offending agent is discontinued. Formaldehyde nail hardeners have been reported as causing onycholysis and also allergic contact dermatitis; they may also act as irritants. Patch testing should be with formaldehyde (1–2% in aqua). Because of its irritant qualities caution should be used in interpreting the reactions.

Stick-on nail dressing, 'press-on' nail polish, synthetic nail covers

Stick-on nail dressings consist of a thin, coloured synthetic film with an adhesive that fixes them firmly to the nail. The pathological changes produced in nails vary considerably in intensity from patient to patient and may include flaking, roughness, ridging, onycholysis, disappearance of the lunula, disorganisation of the nail plate, delaminated and broken nails, mild paronychial inflammation, and often disappearance of the cuticle. In some instances the nail only returns to normal after a year. The effects on the nail are traumatic and not allergic.

Nail-mending kits

These include paper strips of a basic film-forming product to create a 'splint' for the partially fractured nail plate.

Nail wrapping

Essentially, in nail wrapping the free edge of each nail is splinted with layers of a fibrous substance, such as cotton-wool, paper, or plastic film, which is fixed with a variety of nitrocellulose glues. After drying, the edge is shaped, and the nail is coated with enamel. The entire procedure is repeated every 2 weeks.

Cuticle removers or softeners

Cuticle removers contain sodium or potassium hydroxide. If they are left in place for more than approximately 20 minutes minor degrees of irritation may result.

Triethanolamine can be a sensitising agent (5% in petrolatum for patch testing). Cuticle removers contain substances such as quaternary ammonium or urea.

Nail cream

This is an ordinary water-in-oil moisturising cream, with low water (30%) and high lipid content. It should be applied after cleaning the hands to prevent or improve brittleness.

Nail whiteners

The function of nail whiteners is to whiten the unenamelled ends of the fingernails. They may be applied by a pencil containing a white pigment and a vehicle such as stearic acid, beeswax and ozokerites.

Nail buffing

Buffing may be indicated for removing small particles of nail debris, this enhancing the lustre and smoothness of the nail plate. Buffing creams, which contain waxes and finely ground pumice, and buffing powders, are abrasive and should not be overused on thin nails.

Nail changes due to cosmetics used at other sites

(1) Onycholysis may occur due to the use of thioglycolate chemical hair removers. The condition usually affects the distal fourth of several nails.

(2) A yellowish discoloration of the nail can be produced when the nitrocellulose reacts with resorcinol in hair tonics.

(3) Extensive external mercury application, such as bleaching agents for the treatment of melasma, causes a metallic greyish discoloration of the nails.

(4) Discoloration of the fingernails has been noted following the use of a chloroxine-containing shampoo for seborrhoeic dermatitis; chloroxine is known to be highly reactive to metals.

Occupational application of cosmetics resulting in nail damage

Trainee hairdressers usually spend the first year shampooing, which may produce nail fragility and onycholysis. Thioglycolates, used in the permanent waving processes, which distort the keratin fibrils, can cause koilonychia. Brownish staining caused by hair dyes is also common in the nails of hairdressers.

Sales people who demonstrate acrylic artificial nails may become sensitised to liquid monomer. Medical personnel already sensitised to liquid monomer can develop a mild contact dermatitis in spite of precautions taken to avoid contact. The latter is somewhat volatile, and the vapour emanating from an open bottle can cause dermatitis in highly sensitised individuals.

Damage from nail instruments

Metal instruments such as a nail file or scissors, wooden or plastic orange sticks, or nail whitener pencils may create acute or chronic injuries in the nail area. Onycholysis may result from using the sharp point for cleaning under the nail plate. Nails, however, are best cleaned with a nail brush and soap, since over-zealous manicure, pushing back the cuticles, may result in white streaks across several nails (Samman, 1977).

Cleaning around the nail with contaminated instruments may lead to acute or chronic paronychia.

According to Brauer (1984), it is not advisable to cut or clip the nail plate since this produces a shearing action that weakens the natural layered structure and promotes fracturing and splitting. An emery board is preferred for shaping the fingernail by filing from the sides of the nail towards the centre.

Evidently there are many possible side-effects to nail cosmetics but, considering the widespread use of cosmetics by the general population, the incidence of adverse reactions is small. This has been confirmed recently by Skog (1980) who recorded only two cases of allergic dermatitis due to nail cosmetics in a total of 41 patients with contact dermatitis seen at a skin clinic in Stockholm serving a population of approximately 250 000 people. One can conclude that misuse of nail *instruments* is potentially far more damaging to the nail apparatus than are the many cosmetic preparations.

References

Baran, R and Schibli, H (1990) Permanent paresthesia to sculptured nails. A distressing problem. *Derm. Clin.* **8** 139

Brauer, E (1984) Cosmetics: The care and adornment of the nail. In *Diseases of the Nail and their Management*, eds Baran, R and Dawber, R P R, pp. 289–302. Oxford: Blackwell Scientific

Fisher, A A and Baran, R (1991) Adverse reaction to acrylate sculptured nails with particular reference to paresthesia. *Amer. J. Contact Derm.* **2** 38

Nater, J P, de Groot, A C and Liem, D H (1985) *Unwanted Effects of Cosmetics and Drugs used in Dermatology 2nd ed*, pp. 337–342. Amsterdam, Oxford, Princeton: Excerpta Medica

Samman, P D (1977) Nail disorders caused by external influences. *J. Soc. Cosm. Chem.* **28** 351

Skog, E (1980) Incidence of cosmetic dermatitis. *Contact Derm.* **61** 449

Further reading

Baran, R (1982) Pathology induced by the application of cosmetics to the nail. In *Principles of Cosmetics for the Dermatologist*, eds Frost, P and Horwitz, S N, pp. 181–184. St Louis, Missouri: Mosby

Scher, R K (1982) Cosmetics and ancillary preparations for the care of nails. *J. Amer. Acad. Derm.* **6** 523–528

Zaias, N (1980) *The Nail in Health and Disease*, p. 666. Lancaster: MTP Press

10

Nail deformities due to trauma

P. D. Samman

A great many nail deformities are the result of trauma, which may affect the nails in many ways. In this chapter, therefore, a number of otherwise unrelated conditions are discussed.

The damage inflicted on the nail may be the result of a single or occasional injury, or it may be the result of constantly repeated minor injuries. The first type is described as acute trauma and produces permanent damage to the nail if the matrix area is injured. Repeated minor injuries are described as chronic trauma.

Acute trauma

Haematomata

These are probably the commonest occasional injuries inflicted on the nail (Fig. 10.1). The amount of damage varies greatly and in severe cases is accompanied by much pain. Whether or not the haemorrhage is immediately apparent depends on the location of the injury. If it is under the exposed nail the bleeding will be immediately apparent but if the injury is below the dorsal nail fold the haemorrhage may not be visible for 2 or 3 days and will then move forward with the growth of the nail.

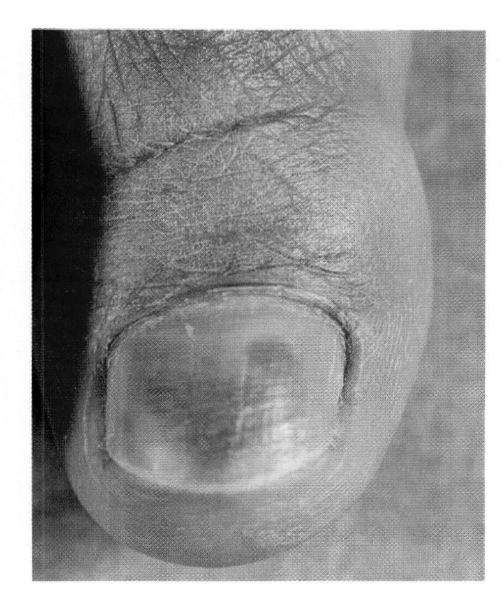

Fig. 10.1 Subungual haematoma

Stone and Mullins (1963) have shown that a haemorrhage in the matrix area is incorporated into the nail plate, while one distal to the lunula remains subcuticular unless removed. In the majority of cases of severe damage, partial or total temporary shedding of the nail occurs if the blood is not released very quickly. Most patients request treatment for the relief of pain. The pain is produced by the increasing pressure below the nail. Reduction of pressure is best carried out by making a small puncture hole through the nail plate with a hot cautery point, or other suitable instrument, without local anaesthesia. This procedure not only relieves the pain but may save the nail. The possibility of an underlying fracture must be considered; in a series described by Farrington (1964) this was present in 19%.

Splits and ridges

Permanent splits will result from any acute trauma which severs the matrix area (Fig. 10.2). The associated injuries are usually more severe and the damage to the nail is not appreciated for some months. It is then observed that the nail is split throughout its length, into two or more portions. If

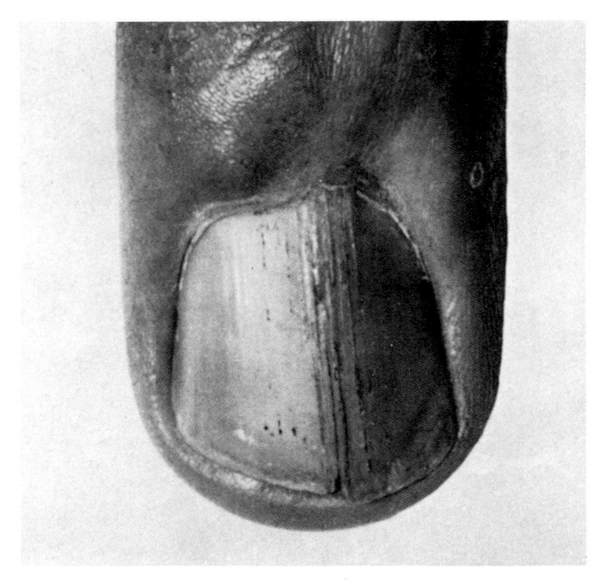

Fig. 10.2 Permanent ridging and splitting of nail following trauma

the damage is reported soon after the injury it may be possible to repair it by removing the nail plate and putting in sutures to pull together the separated parts of the matrix. If successful, the split will be replaced by a ridge down the nail. Unfortunately, it is often not for some months or years after the injury that the damage is reported. In these cases plastic repair may be possible by removing permanently the smaller portion and recentring the remainder (see Johnson, 1971). Sometimes the patient has difficulty in recalling the accident which may have appeared quite minor at the time, but proved sufficient to produce permanent damage to the matrix.

Permanent ridges on isolated nails are produced by similar injuries to those producing splits, but of lesser degree.

Pigment bands

Bands of pigmentation may often form in the nail plate after minor injuries in patients with heavily pigmented skin. A sewing machine needle run through the finger at the level of the nail matrix is readily recalled by the patient (Fig. 10.3), but much less damage may produce the same effect. The resulting pigment bands may be temporary or permanent. In the white races, bands of pigment appear on the nail plate much less often and in these people may be the result of an active junctional naevus in the matrix area (p. 176).

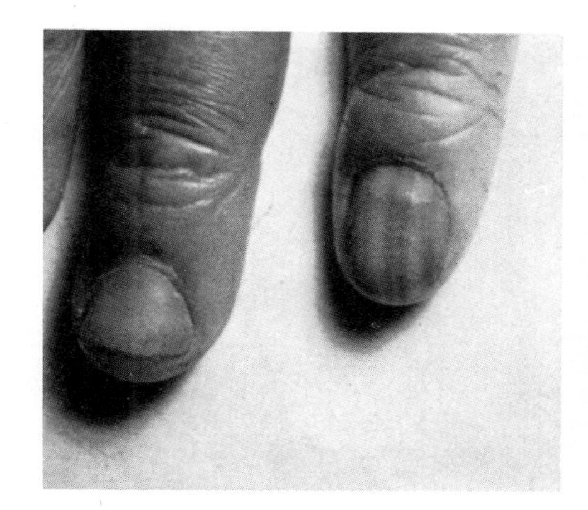

Fig. 10.3 Pigmented bands on nail plate following injury with sewing machine needle

Other deformities

It is not uncommon to see a patient with a partially amputated fingertip with a severely distorted nail often short and thick, the end result of an injury to the finger. Great hypertrophy of the nail is occasionally the result of a single injury but more often is the result of repeated trauma (p. 164).

Chronic trauma

It will be seen that there are several ways in which repeated trauma may be inflicted. Nail biting, cuticle biting, and playing with the nails or cuticles are all common habits which may produce considerable damage to the nails. Ill-fitting footwear, especially in children, will lead to many nail deformities of the toes (Fig. 10.4). Injuries from chemicals or friction at work or in the home may result in damage in various ways (Fig. 10.5), while the use of nail varnish may occasionally produce

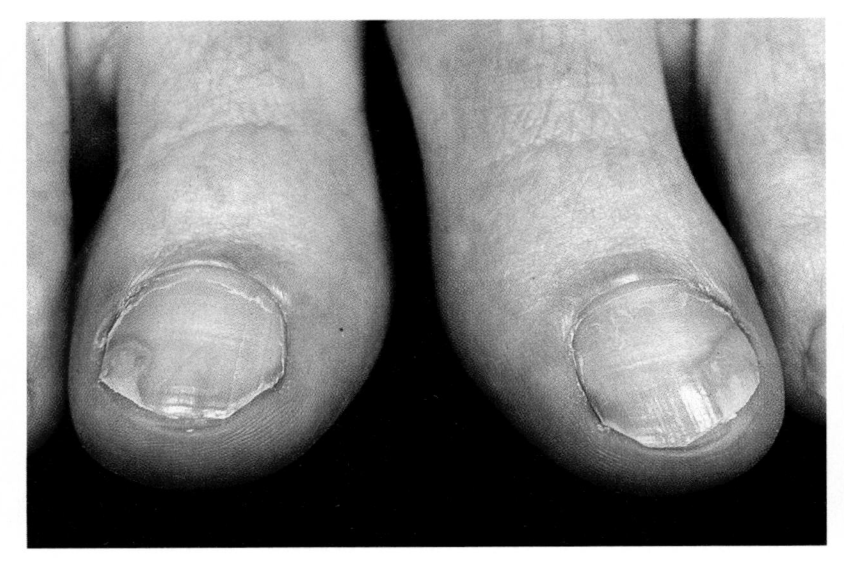

Fig. 10.4 Traumatic onycholysis from wearing tight shoes

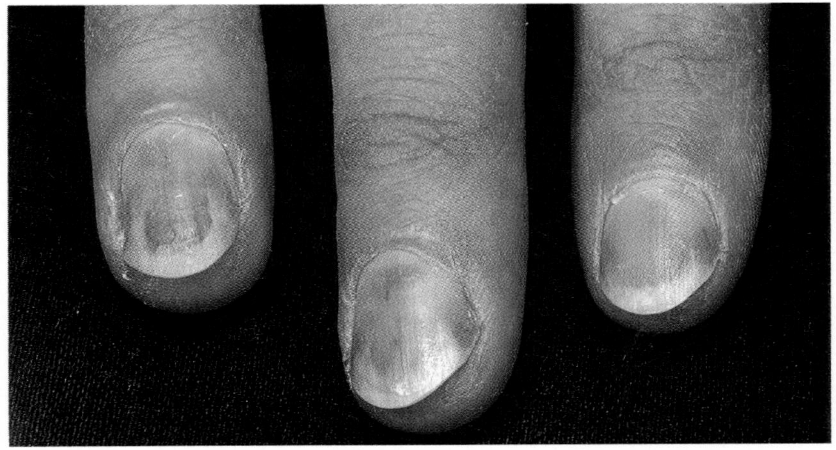

Fig. 10.5 Traumatic onycholysis from guitar playing

staining of the nails which cannot easily be removed. Frequent immersion of the hands in water is a more subtle form of injury but is probably the most important factor in the splitting of the nail into layers.

Nail biting and cuticle biting

These very common habits may produce great distortion of the nail. Patients will usually freely admit to the habit but occasionally will claim that the deformity is due to lack of growth of the nail. This can easily be disproved by putting a fixed dressing on one finger for a few weeks or by making a small mark on one nail near the half-moon and watching it move to the tip a few weeks later. Bitten nails, which are usually very short and irregular, in fact are said to grow rather faster than normal (Fig. 10.6). The patient spends much time biting off spicules formed at an earlier session of biting. Cuticle biting is similar and may result in recurrent attacks of paronychia usually of a minor nature. Some people may bite only one nail and then only in times of stress such as watching an exciting television programme. The biting in these cases may be away from the tip and may even encroach

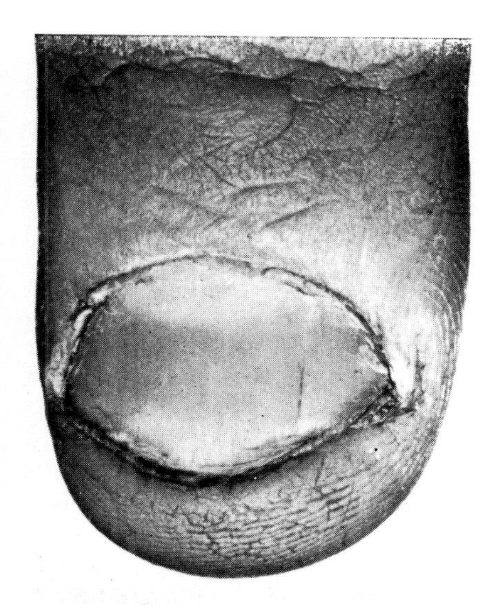

Fig. 10.6 Bitten nail

on the matrix area, when an entirely different deformity will be produced (Fig. 10.7). If the damage produced by biting is severe the patient may further aggravate the condition by picking off small pieces constantly so that there may be apparent total loss of the nail. An occlusive dressing applied to the finger tip will prevent further damage and permit regrowth of a normal nail (Samman, 1977). In any case of nail deformity otherwise unexplained, it is always worth enquiring about nail biting. Rarely, the reverse occurs and one nail is spared while the remainder are bitten.

Deformities very similar to nail biting can be caused by picking at the nail or by very close trimming.

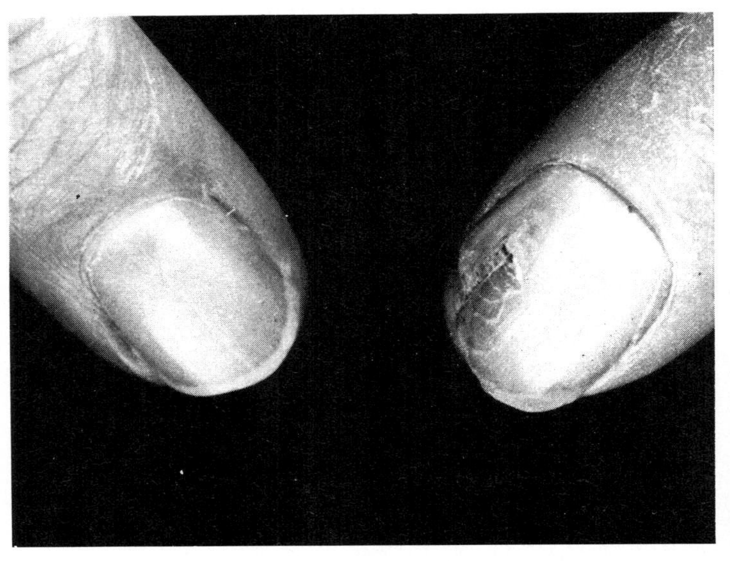

Fig. 10.7 Bitten nail—damage due to biting over matrix area

Treatment of nail biting is very unsatisfactory. The answer is obvious, but the patient often cannot be persuaded to give up the habit. If one parent nail bites, the children are more likely to be nail biters than otherwise and it may prove more easy to reason with the parent than with the child. Periungual warts are an important complication of nail biting, and treatment of these is discussed on p. 169.

Hang nails

Hang nails are very common in nail biters but may also result from many other forms of injury incurred in the home or at work. They consist of small portions of horny epidermis which have split away from the lateral nail fold. They may extend deep enough to expose the underlying cutis when they will be painful and may be the site of origin of bacterial infection. They are best treated by cutting away with very sharp pointed scissors. If infection is present, an antiseptic paint should be applied.

The habit tic of playing with the nails

This is another, but less common, habit (Samman, 1963) and often produces a rather characteristic deformity (Fig. 10.8). The damage is usually inflicted on one or both thumb nails by one of the fingers of the same hand. The finger is placed on the dorsal nail fold and then drawn forward over the nail plate (Fig. 10.9) and the process is repeated frequently. The damage is caused partly by this and partly by picking at the cuticle. The cuticle will be seen to be pulled away from the nail (Macaulay, 1966).

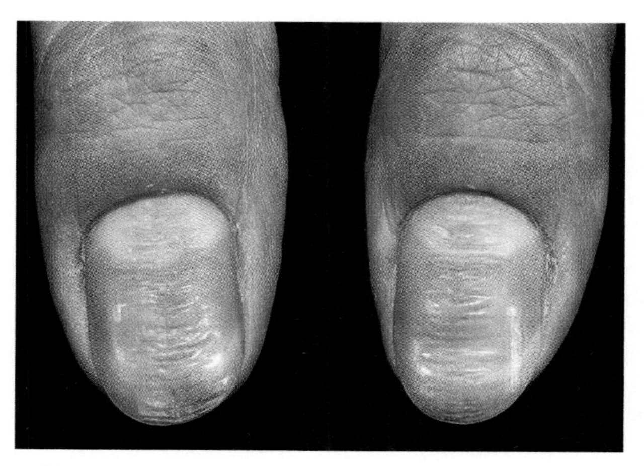

Fig. 10.8 Traumatic nail dystrophy due to habit tic

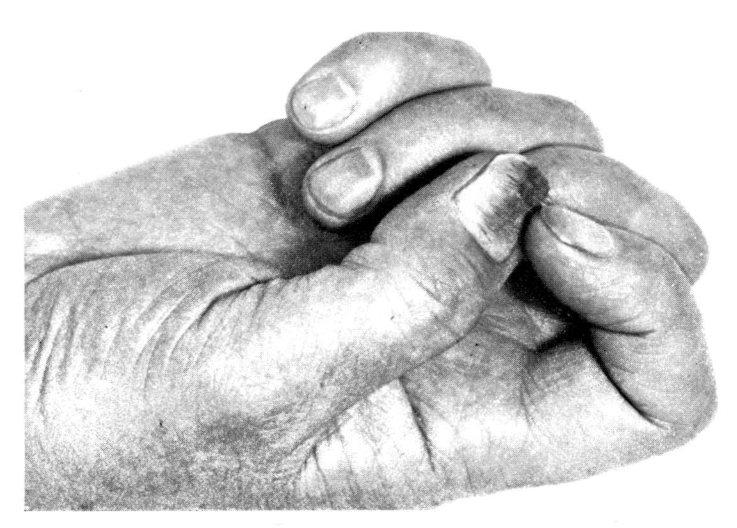

Fig. 10.9 Habit tic—method of formation

Less often, a finger of the opposite hand is used to pick at the cuticle. The resulting damage usually takes the form of a depression about 2 mm wide down the centre of the nail from the cuticle to the tip, from which extend a number of cross-ridges almost to the edges of the nail. The depression is not always present and may be seen on one thumb nail but not on the other. When the depression is absent, the cross-ridging is the only visible sign. The presence or absence of a depression probably depends on the force used by the finger which produces the damage. In a few cases a finger other than the thumb carries the deformity and in these cases it is the thumb which does the damage. The patient is usually well aware of his habit tic, but is surprised when the cause of his deformity is explained to him.

The only conditions likely to be mistaken for this deformity are true median dystrophy (dystrophia mediana canaliformis of Heller) which is described on p. 99, dermatitis affecting the nail and trauma inflicted by other means. In dermatitis the cross-ridges are less regular than in the habit tic and there is likely to be evidence of dermatitis on the finger or a recent history of dermatitis. In median dystrophy there is a true split down the nail and the lateral projections are of a feathery appearance. Occasionally cross-ridging is the result of over active pushing back of the cuticle during manicuring, or it may be the result of repeated intense pressure on the tip of the nail.

The condition will correct itself if the patient gives up the habit or if an occlusive dressing is applied over the affected finger for a sufficient time.

Damage to nails in mushroom growers

Schubert *et al.* (1977) describe five cases of damage to the finger nails in patients working on mushroom beds. The damage consisted of koilonychia, usure des ongles, onycholysis, longitudinal splitting and some splinter haemorrhages. The traumatic cause was due to repeated rubbing of nails in workers lifting heavy plastic bags.

Nutcracker's nails

This title was used to describe nail splitting and onycholysis in a patient who separated the two halves of cracked walnuts with his nails over a period of 10 years (Cohen, Lewis and Resnik, 1975).

Onychotillomania (Figs. 10.10, 10.11, 10.12)

A few cases of this deformity have been seen by the author. It was described by Combes and Scott (1951). Essentially it is similar to the habit tic but aetiologically is closer to parasitophobia. The patient picks off small pieces of nail and fragments of skin from the surrounding nail fold and may claim that they contain parasites. A rough and irregular nail and nail fold results. Many finger nails are involved.

Nail artefacts

These fortunately are rare. They are produced by deliberate trauma and take various forms. Piercing the nail with a sharp instrument in the region of the half-moon interferes with nail

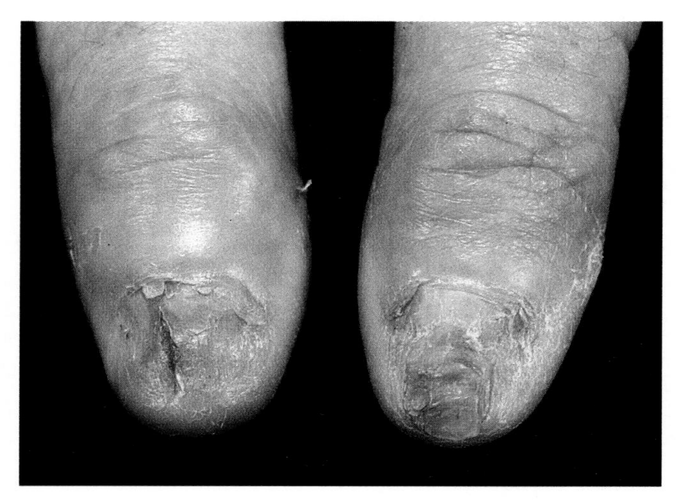

Fig. 10.10 Onychotillomania—thumb nails

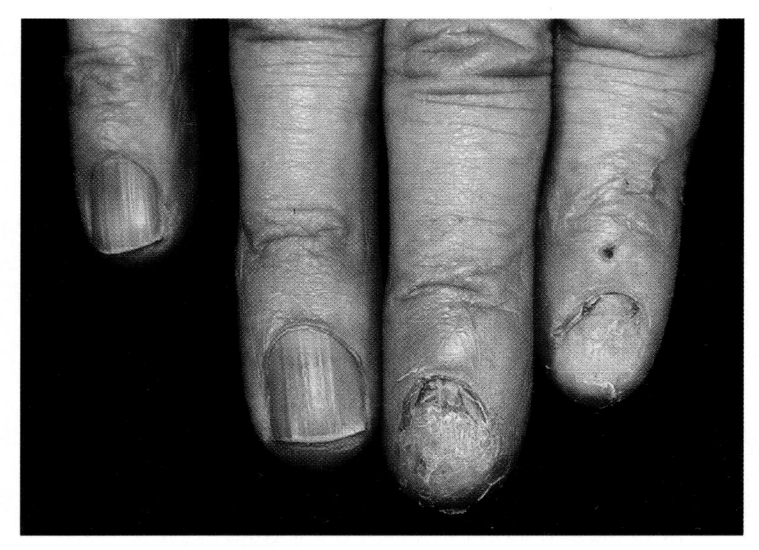

Fig. 10.11 Onychotillomania—finger nails

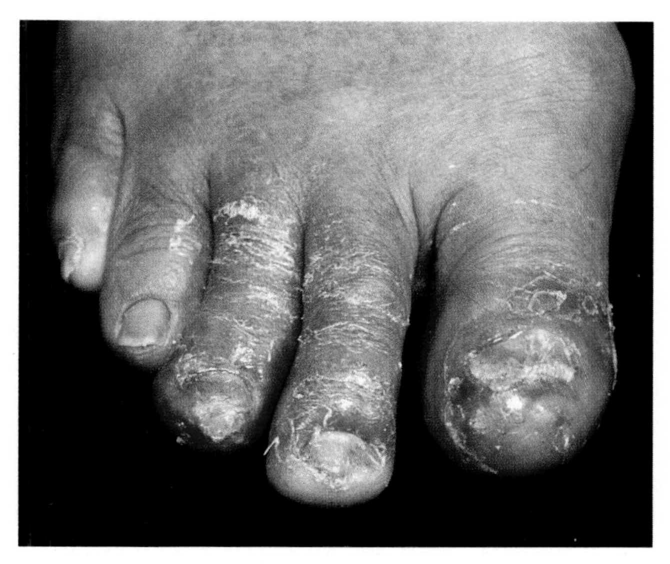

Fig. 10.12 Onychotillomania—toe nails

growth locally and, as a result of sepsis, granulation tissue may project through the nail. In another form the patient inserts a nail file or other instrument under the cuticle and by so doing produces a chronic or acute paronychia (Fig. 10.13). Several fingers or toes may be involved. The patient will gain some benefit from the injury.

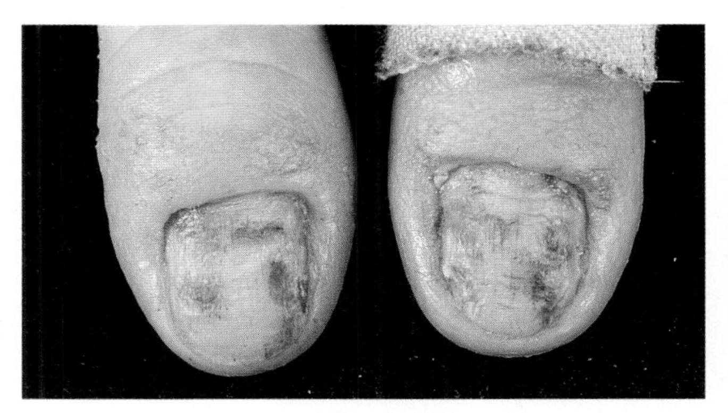

Fig. 10.13 Deliberately produced nail haemorrhage and paronychia

Splitting into layers (lamellar dystrophy)

This is a very common complaint among women. The nails do not split along ridges longitudinally but horizontally through the thickness of the nail so that portions of the surface break off near the free margin (Fig. 10.14). Many forms of trauma probably contribute to the cause of this complaint, but the most important may be the repeated uptake and drying out of water.

When immersed in water, especially if alkaline, the nail quickly becomes soft through the taking up of excess water, but this excess is quickly lost again on exposure to a dry atmosphere. This repeated wetting and drying leads to a lack of adhesion between the cells of the nail plate and splits develop. These splits can easily be shown to exist microscopically before the patient becomes aware of the damage they may cause. Although common in women, this condition is seldom seen in men. There are probably a number of reasons why this is so: first, women like to keep their nails longer than men so that there is more free margin with both surfaces exposed to the atmosphere and therefore wetting and drying occur more rapidly; second, women more often have their hands in water than men; third, nail varnish and varnish removers and excess manicuring may be of some importance aetiologically; and, finally, women are more conscious of their nails than men and are therefore more likely to report the defect. The condition is more common in winter than in summer, probably because in winter the atmosphere is drier.

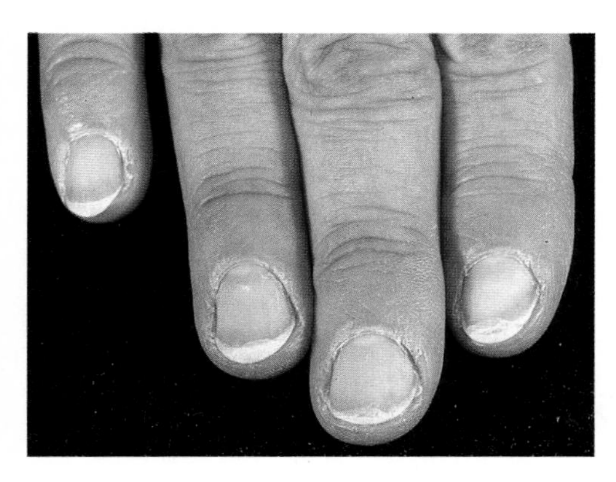

Fig. 10.14 Splitting of nail into layers

Shelley and Shelley (1984) have done a scanning electron microscopic study of clippings from the tips of affected nails and from controls. The electronmicrograph of affected nails showed over 30 laminar splits of the leading edge, each lamina being one cell thick. A cross-section of nails 2 mm from the tip showed fault lines which were not present in controls. The authors suggest that the cell separation results from a failure of intercellular cement substance to hold when subjected to ordinary trauma such as acetone to remove varnish, and detergents.

Treatment is unfortunately unsatisfactory. The patient should be instructed to avoid excess wetting as far as possible and to keep her nails as short as she will tolerate. Nail varnish should not be forbidden because this at least covers the defect to some extent. Oily removers should, however, be recommended. The author has not found calcium or gelatin to be of any real value in treatment. A good nail hardener is needed but one that is free from irritants or sensitisers such as formaldehyde.

Very occasionally a single nail is encountered which is split into two layers throughout its length (Fig. 10.15). This is different from lamellar dystrophy and is the result of a

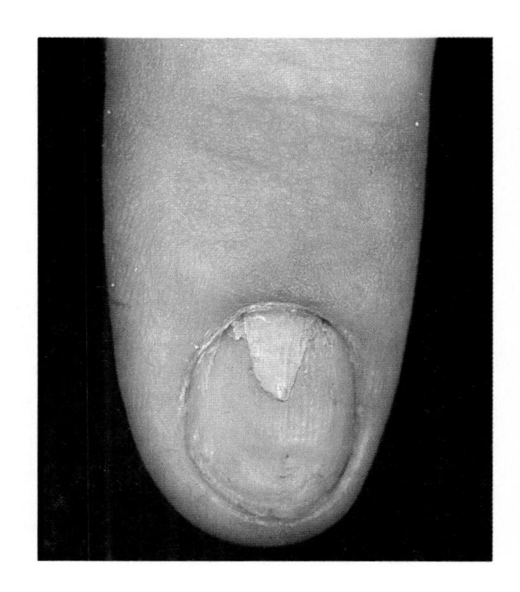

Fig. 10.15 Trauma has split nail into two layers

single injury splitting the matrix. This is sometimes called *onychoschizia*.

Cutaneous microwave injury

Under this heading Brodkin and Bleiberg (1975) described nail deformities in two patients who were operating a microwave oven which was probably faulty. The damage consisted of deep cross-ridges on the nails of the fingers which opened and closed the oven. The patients suffered no discomfort.

Damage caused by footwear

Ingrowing toe nails

Although the aetiology of ingrowing toe nails is disputed there seems no doubt that trauma is the major factor in their causation. In the first place unsatisfactory footwear leads to deformities of the feet, then incorrect cutting of the toe nails produces spicules of nail which inflict damage to the lateral nail folds. The great toe nails are most often affected and these suffer the greatest damage during locomotion. Hyperhidrosis is an aggravating factor.

In the early stages there is discomfort and slight local sepsis (Fig. 10.16) but as the condition progresses granulation tissue forms in the lateral nail fold, the infection becomes more severe and pain more intense. The majority of cases are produced by spicules of nail penetrating the lateral nail fold. In time, the spicule separates to a large extent from the main part of the nail and, being embedded in the soft tissues of the lateral nail fold, acts as a foreign body. Some cases are due to over-curvature of the nail when increasing pressure results in damage to the nail fold. A few cases develop during the treatment of fungal infection of the finger nail with griseofulvin. The toe nails which are also diseased have become shrunken and the nail bed is also reduced in size. When treatment with griseofulvin is begun the condition of the toe nails improves to some extent, sufficiently to produce a nail which is wider than can be accommodated by the shrunken nail bed. Many treatments for this condition have been

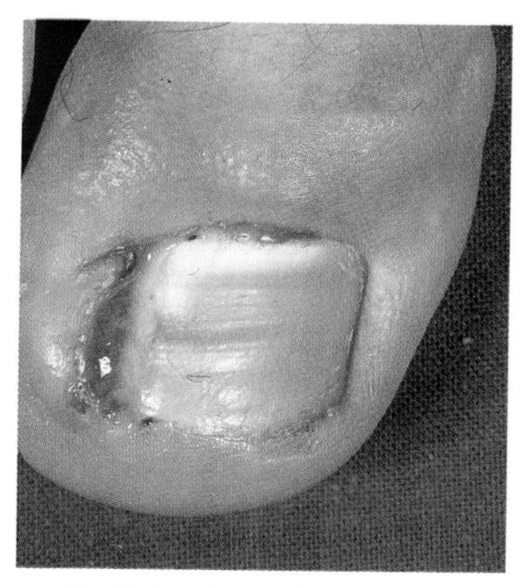

Fig. 10.16 Ingrowing toe nails

recommended. Lloyd-Davies and Brill (1963) have shown that conservative treatment is to be recommended in most cases. They say that the patient must be instructed in foot care and sensible shoes must be worn. The nails should be cut at right angles to their long axis leaving well-defined corners. Treatment consists of soaking the feet in warm water twice daily followed by careful drying and the application of a foot powder; caking of the powder must be avoided. A small quantity of cotton wool is then introduced gently under the corners of the nail, the patient being shown how to do this. Granulation tissue is cauterised with silver nitrate (in the outpatient department). It is essential, however, that any spicule which has penetrated the nail fold be removed or continuing infection will result. This may require careful dissection to locate and remove the spicule.

With this method of treatment, cure is usually obtained in about 6 weeks. Operation is reserved for patients who fail to respond to conservative measures, for patients who have had the condition for a long time and demand operation, or when there is cellulitis or severe pain. For details of surgical treatment see p. 219.

Very occasionally finger or thumb nails become ingrowing. In these cases there may be no apparent trauma. Management is similar to that for toe nails.

Excess curvature in the long axis of the nail also usually affects the great toe nails. Although it may produce an ingrowing nail, sometimes it causes great discomfort from partial strangulation of the soft tissues of the distal phalanx without breaking the epidermis. Cornelius and Shelley (1968) call this type of injury the pincer nail syndrome. Treatment should consist of removal of the nail plate.

Excess curvature may also be found occasionally in psoriasis and on other occasions without apparent cause. The condition may affect finger (especially thumb) (Fig. 10.17) or toe nails and several may be involved. Some will come to look like claws.

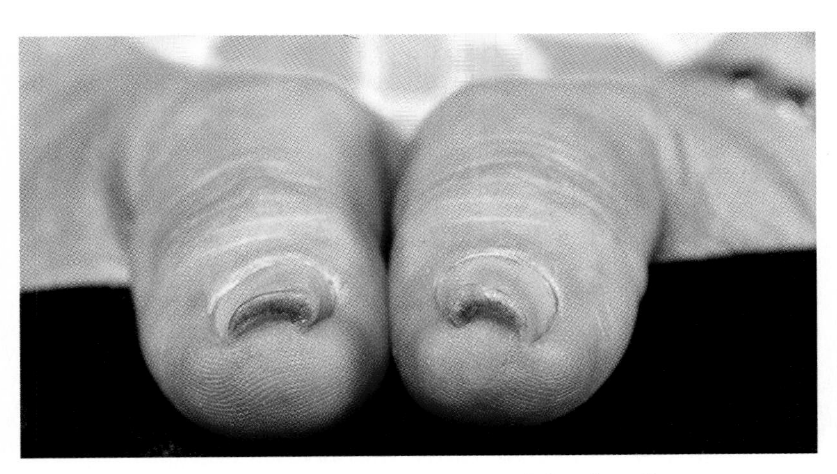

Fig. 10.17 Excessive curvature of thumb nails

Onychogryphosis and hypertrophied nails

In this group of disorders trauma is only one factor in its causation and some cases are probably developmental (Fig. 10.18). The fact that trauma can produce hypertrophy of the nail was well illustrated by one patient, who could accurately date the commencement of the enlargement to a single injury some years previously. Onychogryphosis was once known as ostler's nail because some cases could be traced to injury caused by a horse trampling on the foot of the ostler while he was shoeing the horse.

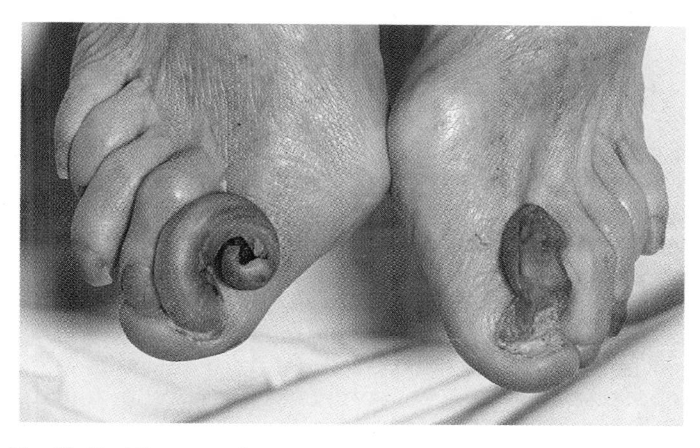

Fig. 10.18 Hypertrophy and onychogryphosis of great toe nails

Onychogryphosis usually affects the great toe nail (Fig. 10.19), but others may also be involved; the nails become thick and curved and are extremely hard to cut so they are left untrimmed by the patient. The longer they grow the

Fig. 10.19 Onychogryphosis

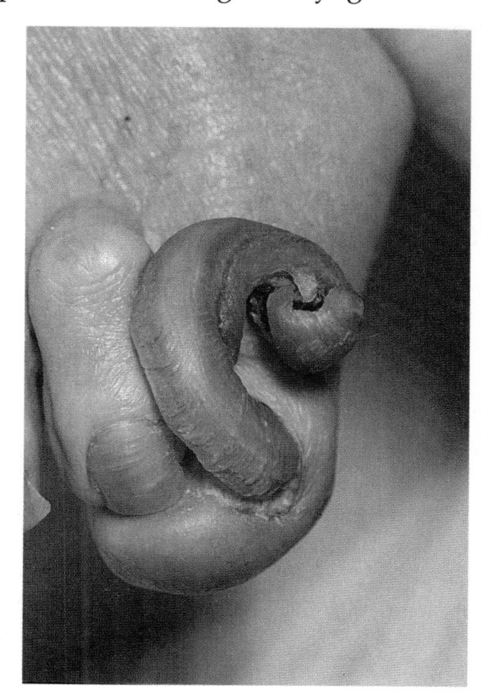

greater the trauma inflicted by footwear so that the damage is progressive.

Nail hypertrophy implies thickening and increase in length while onychogryphosis implies curvature so that the nail resembles a ram's horn. Other causes of nail hypertrophy are given on p. 24.

Treatment is difficult and can be either radical or palliative. In elderly subjects palliative treatment is preferred and consists of regular paring of the affected nails. This will usually be carried out by a chiropodist using nail clippers and a file, or a mechanical burr. Not infrequently the nail is invaded by granulation tissue from the nail bed and cutting into this will cause pain and haemorrhage. In younger persons the nail may be removed from time to time and allowed to regrow. The process is repeated when necessary or the nail may be permanently removed by destruction of the matrix. The latter procedure does, however, produce a rather unstable toe and the less destructive measure is often preferred even though it needs to be repeated occasionally.

Shedding of the toe nails

Even quite minor injury such as the wearing for a few hours of shoes which are too short may result in the formation of a subungual haematoma and this may progress to the loss of the nail some weeks later. The nail will, of course, be replaced in time. The great toe nails may be shed periodically in some persons, for example footballers, as a result of repeated minor injuries even in the absence of a haematoma. The condition is probably restricted to persons with some underlying instability. Oliver (1927) described the condition in three members of a family. At times, anatomical features such as an unusually long great toe may contribute to the cause. No treatment is needed but the probable cause should be explained to the patient.

Many cases of subungual haematoma of one or both great toe nails with or without actual nail loss have been encountered in patients wearing platform shoes (Fig. 10.20). This was first noted by Almeyda (1973). The platform shoe is too rigid and during walking causes repeated minor trauma to the nail. A change to a peep-toe type of platform shoe should prevent recurrence.

Familial periodic shedding is discussed on p. 197.

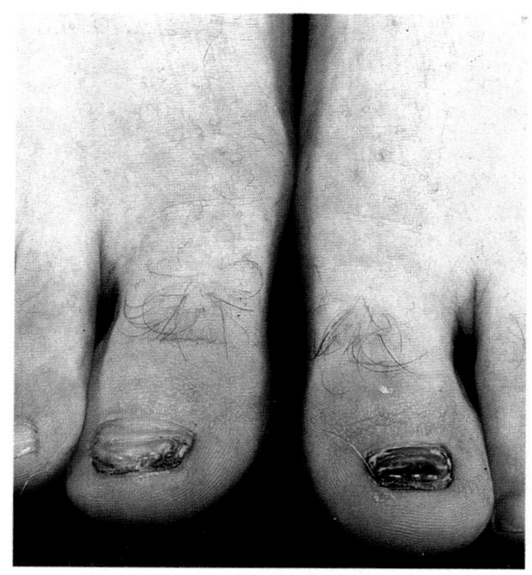

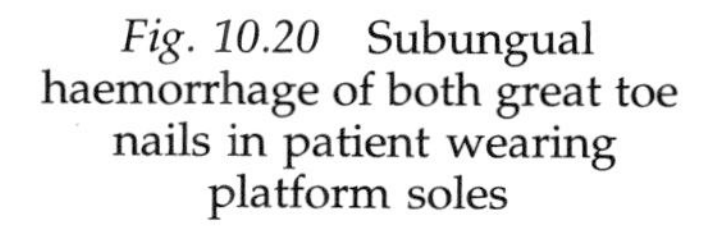

Fig. 10.20 Subungual haemorrhage of both great toe nails in patient wearing platform soles

Worn-down toe nails

Occasionally patients complain that some of their toe nails do not grow and it is apparent that they are being worn down by constant rubbing against the shoe. The condition is harmless and an explanation is all that is required for treatment.

References

Almeyda, J (1973) Platform nails (letter). *Brit. Med. J.* **1** 176

Brodkin, R H, and Bleiberg, J (1975) Cutaneous microwave injury. *Acta Dermatovenereol.* **53** 50

Cohen, B H, Lewis, L A and Resnik, S S (1975) Nutcracker's nails. *Cutis* **16** 141

Combes, F C and Scott, M J (1951) Onychotillomania. *Arch. Derm.* **63** 778

Cornelius, C and Shelley, W B (1968) Pincer nail syndrome. *Arch. Surg.* **96** 321

Farrington, G H (1964) Subungual haematoma—an evaluation of treatment. *Brit. Med. J.* **1** 742

Johnson, R K (1971) Nailplasty. *Plast. Reconstr. Surg.* **47** 275

Lloyd-Davies, R W and Brill, G G (1963) The aetiology and outpatient management of ingrowing toe nails. *Brit. J. Surg.* **50** 592

Macaulay, W L (1966) Transverse ridging of the thumb nails. *Arch. Derm.* **93** 421

Oliver, W J (1927) Recurrent onychoptosis occurring as a family disorder. *Brit. J. Derm.* **39** 297

Samman, P D (1963) A traumatic nail dystrophy produced by a habit tic. *Arch. Derm.* **88** 895

Samman, P D (1977) Nail disorders caused by external influences. *J. Soc. Cosm. Chem.* **28** 351

Schubert, B, Minard, J J, Baran, R *et al.* (1977) Onycopathy of mushroom growers. *Ann. Derm. Syph.* **104** 627

Shelley, W B and Shelley, E D (1984) Onychoschizia. Scanning electron microscopy. *J. Amer. Acad. Derm.* **10** 623

Stone, O J and Mullins, J F (1963) The distal course of nail matrix haemorrhage. *Arch. Derm.* **88** 186

11

Tumours producing nail disorders

P. D. Samman

Benign tumours

Warts

By far the commonest tumour to develop near the nail is the wart. When growing below the nail plate it often penetrates deeply like a plantar wart, but around the nail it resembles more closely the common wart of other parts of the dorsum of the hand. Not infrequently it involves the whole of the nail fold. It is a frequent complication of nail biting (Fig. 11.1). The nail plate itself is only occasionally affected by the warts. It may be displaced upwards by warts under the nails and at times becomes irregular from the presence of periungual warts. Most of the damage to the nail is due to the associated nail biting. Patients almost invariably report for treatment of the warts and not for abnormalities of the nail.

It is often said that treatment of warts near the nail is difficult but generally they respond as well to conventional methods as do most multiple warts. Treatment with electrocautery or diathermy under local anaesthesia is the method of choice for adults but in young children the author prefers to use a combination of monochloracetic acid and 40% salicylic acid plaster. This method of treatment was detailed by Halpern

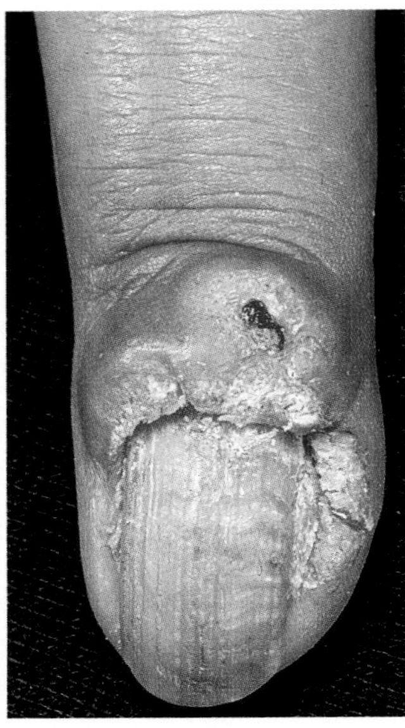

Fig. 11.1 Periungual warts

and Lane (1953). A saturated solution of monochloracetic acid is applied to the wart by a wisp of cotton wool around the end of an orange stick. When dry it is covered with 40% salicylic acid plaster cut to the size of the wart and this is held in place by two or three layers of zinc oxide adhesive tape. The patient is instructed to remove the plasters after 3 days and to apply a light dressing if necessary. The patient is seen again after 7–14 days when many of the warts may be picked out or the treatment repeated if necessary. At the first visit the acid should be applied rather sparingly, as keratin will take up a considerable quantity if allowed to do so. A too-liberal application will result in pus formation and pain, but no permanent damage to the nail fold, which shows remarkable powers of regeneration. It is usually unnecessary to pare down the wart before the acid is applied. Unlike trichloracetic acid, monochloracetic acid does not whiten the skin when applied.

For warts below the nail it is necessary to cut away the overlying nail before treatment is started. Again electrocautery or diathermy is often the method of choice but the author has found that a number of these will respond to 3% formalin. The fingertip is held in the formalin solution for 10–15 minutes daily for 14–21 days. If the wart does not harden and die within this time it is unwise to continue as formalin dermatitis may develop.

Periungual fibroma

Fibromata growing from the nail fold are frequent stigmata of adenoma sebaceum but are at times seen without other evidence of this disorder (Figs. 11.2, 11.3). They cause little real disability but give rise to some inconvenience and at times may be the cause of a depression forming on the nail plate.

The diagnosis is usually obvious and treatment is by excision if requested. Histologically they may show vascular lakes near the tip (Pardo-Castello and Pardo, 1960).

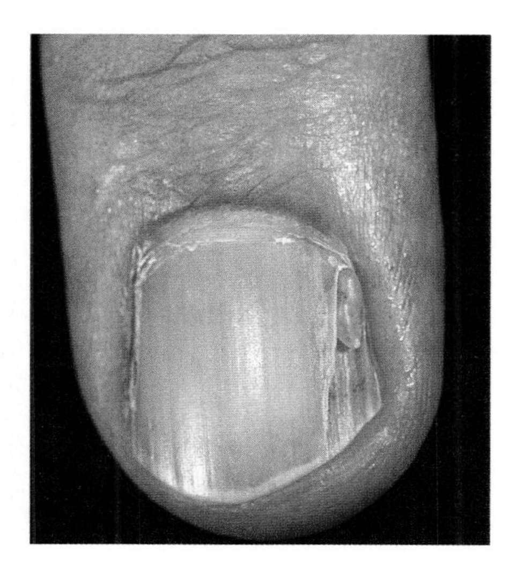

Fig. 11.2 Periungual fibroma

Garlic clove fibroma

Under this heading, Steel (1965) described a small tumour growing away from the nail bed and projecting from the cuticle over the finger or toe. It is loosely attached by a pedicle. The tumour is either a benign epitheliomatous polyp or an irritation fibroma of the nail bed. Histological examination

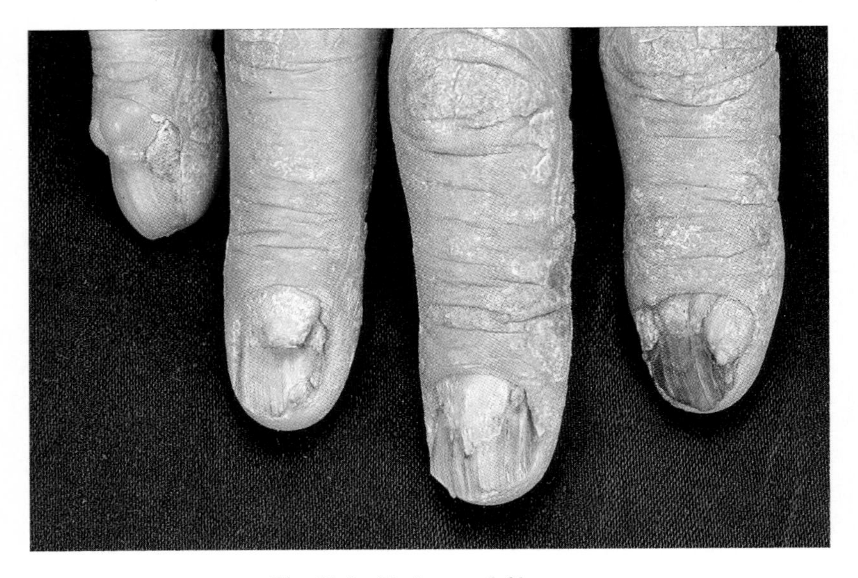

Fig. 11.3 Periungual fibroma

shows that it is covered, except at its base, by a layer of stratified squamous epithelium. The core is composed of interlacing bundles of dense collagenous tissue with capillary channels. Treatment is by excision. Undeutsch and Shrieferstein (1974) describe a similar condition under the heading of garlic corm fibroma. Cahn (1977) has reviewed the cases of garlic clove and garlic corm fibroma in association with a case of his own and reports that they are the same as cases described by Bart *et al.* (1968) as acquired digital fibrokeratoma. Cahn prefers the name 'acquired periungual fibrokeratoma' for the nail cases and says the condition is a distinct clinical and histopathological entity and is reactive hyperplasia initiated by trauma. Kikuchi, Ishii and Inque (1978) also describe a case and show clearly that it arises in the dermis proximal to the nail matrix.

A small filamentous tumour growing below the nail and extending the whole length of the nail plate has been seen by the author on a number of occasions. It presents at the tip of the digit below the nail and can be traced under the nail plate to the cuticle. The nail may be slightly ridged over it. The nosology of this tumour has not yet been determined but it may be a subungual fibroma. It normally causes no trouble so that treatment is not required. It pares down painlessly when the nail is cut.

Subungual exostosis

This is not uncommon and is most often seen on the great toes. It presents as a firm swelling below the nail near the tip and in time will displace the nail (Figs. 11.4, 11.5); it is often mistaken for a wart. X-ray will establish the diagnosis in every case (Fig. 11.6) (Evison, 1966). It is not a true exostosis but an outgrowth

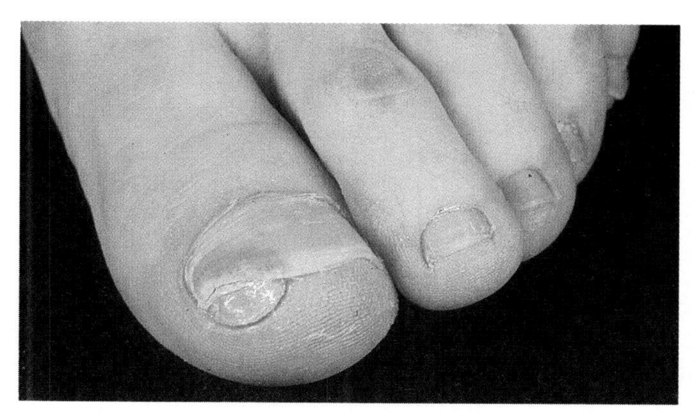

Fig. 11.4 Subungual exostosis

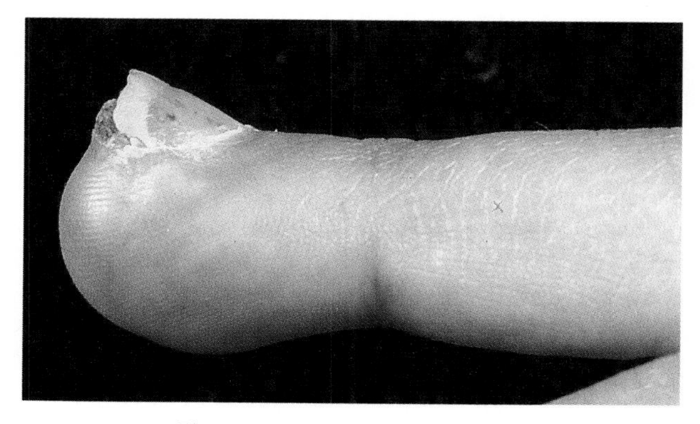

Fig. 11.5 Subungual exostosis

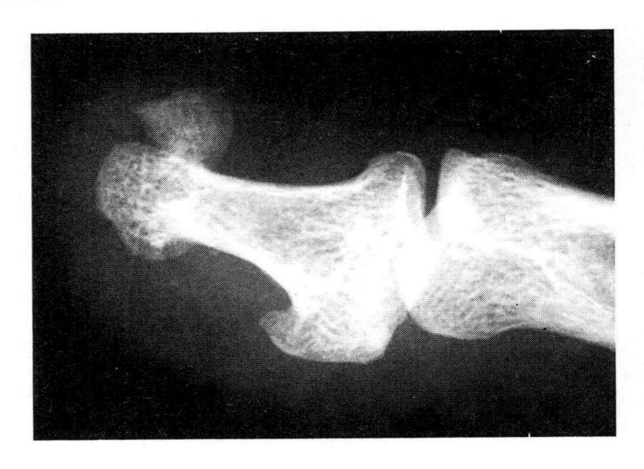

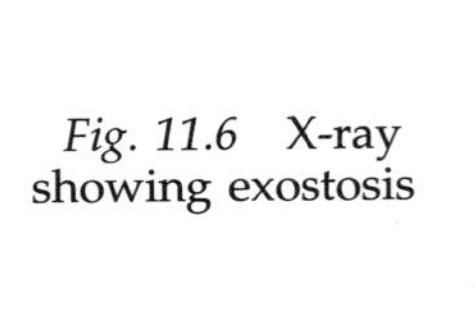

Fig. 11.6 X-ray showing exostosis

of normal bone. Treatment is by excision with strict aseptic precautions because the outgrowth from the distal phalanx must be cut away.

Subungual osteochondroma

Under this heading Appelberg *et al.* (1979) describe five cases of a condition which they say differs from an exostosis because it is commoner in females than males while the reverse is true for exostosis. It consists of a circumscribed pedunculated or sessile bony growth seen on X-ray to be projecting from the dorsum of the distal phalanx. It may be congenital but normally presents at age 10–25 and starts to grow before or at puberty. It has a long slow growth and distorts the nail.

Mucous cyst

This is not a true tumour but a collagenous degeneration of the extensor tendon presenting as a tumour; it has often in the past been designated as a synovial cyst. The condition almost always forms on the dorsum of the distal phalanx between the distal interphalangeal joint and the base of the nail. It is usually quite small (Fig. 11.7), but occasionally quite large (Fig. 11.8). It frequently deforms the nail by producing a depression, 1–2 mm across, throughout the length

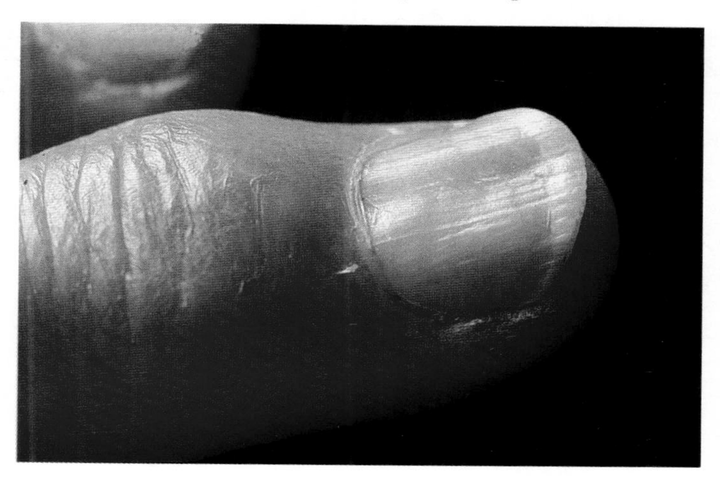

Fig. 11.7 Mucous cyst producing depression in nail plate

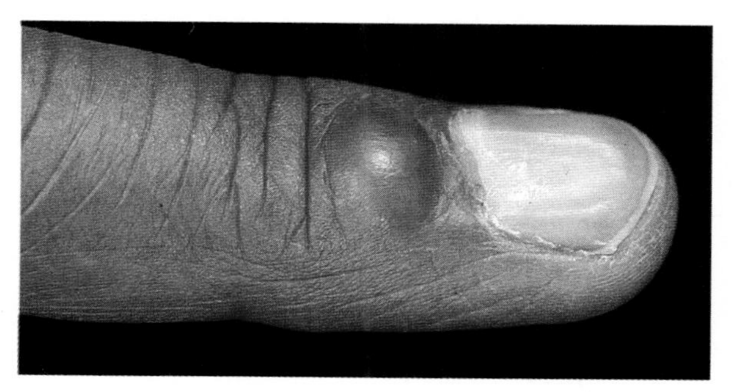

Fig. 11.8 Mucous cyst—large lesion

of the nail. A small quantity of the contents of the cyst escapes down the groove below the cuticle from time to time (Fig. 11.9). The lesion often accompanies osteoarthritis of the adjacent interphalangeal joint.

Except for the nail deformity, the condition is harmless, but if it is deforming the nail or is unsightly because of its size it should be excised (Arner, Lindholm and Romanus, 1956) or a few drops of a depot steroid (such as methylprednisolone) may be injected. No treatment is perfect and the condition may relapse even after excision.

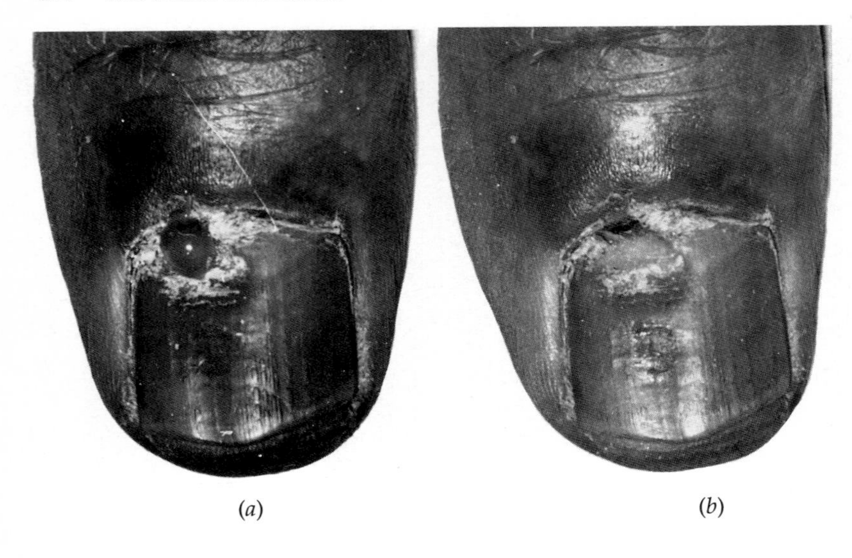

(*a*) (*b*)

Fig. 11.9(a) and (b) Fluid escaping from mucous cyst

Glomus tumour

This is a rare tumour which may develop in the corium of the nail bed giving rise to great pain. The pain may be spontaneous or occur with pressure. The lesion is minute but can usually be seen through the nail plate as a bluish discoloration. It arises from hypertrophy of a glomus body. Treatment should consist of total excision with full aseptic precautions. If not completely removed, recurrence is probable.

Pigmented naevus

In Caucasians a longitudinal band of pigment in the nail plate may be due to a junctional naevus in the nail matrix (Harvey, 1960) (Fig. 11.10). The effect is due to a spill of pigment into the nail plate. It may start at any age, but once it begins it tends to persist indefinitely. These lesions have been known to become malignant, so for lesions on the toe nails and the less important finger nails it is wise to recommend removal of the nail followed by excision of the affected area of the matrix and suture of the cut edges. This procedure will leave a ridge or

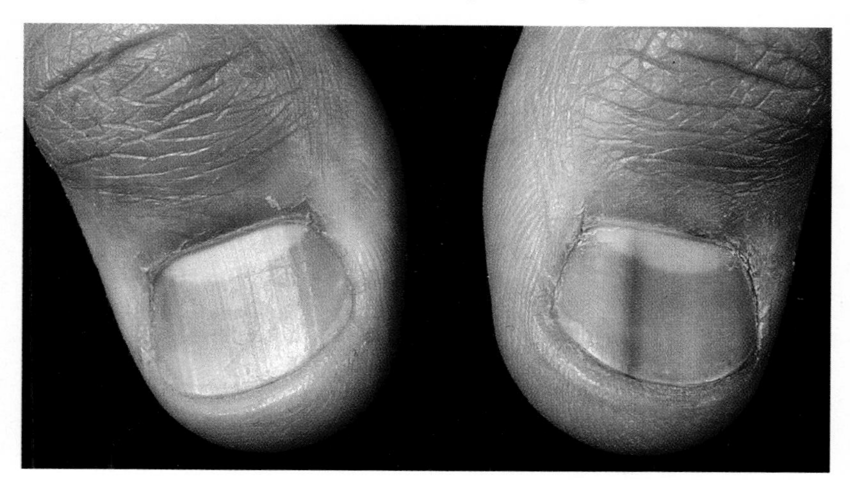

Fig. 11.10 Pigmented band due to junctional naevus

even a permanent split in the nail when it regrows, so for the thumb and index finger a policy of wait and watch is justified.

Pigment streaks in the nails in black people are much more common and are due to minor trauma (p. 150).

Enchondroma

This tumour is very rarely encountered in the distal phalanx when it may present either as chronic paronychia (Shelley and Ralston, 1964) or with greater distortion of the nail (Yaffee, 1965). X-rays will show a radiolucent defect with expansion of the distal phalanx. Treatment is by removal of the chondroid tissue and by filling the cavity so formed with a bone graft if necessary. The condition must be distinguished from an epithelioma or a malignant melanoma which may present in the same way.

Keratoacanthoma

This tumour is relatively common on the face and diagnosis is easily established but, when occurring below the nail, is uncommon and quite unlike the classical lesion (Lamp *et al.*,

1964). It presents as redness and swelling of the tips of the digit with increasing pain. For a few weeks progress is rapid and it may mimic chronic paronychia. Part of the nail separates from the nail bed and a crusted nodule appears at the edge. X-ray shows extensive destruction of the distal phalanx. Histologically it is the same as in the classical lesion and may easily be mistaken for an epithelioma. Stoll and Ackerman (1980) point out that in this location it is a special type of keratoacanthoma which does not regress spontaneously. It is more destructive than a squamous carcinoma in this area. Treatment is by excision after removal of the overlying nail, but partial amputation is not required.

Pyogenic granuloma

A classical pyogenic granuloma near the nail is somewhat rare but if it occurs it should be removed with curette and cautery.

As a malignant melanoma may present in this way, this possibility must be considered.

Excess granulation tissue simulating a pyogenic granuloma is much more common, especially in relation to an ingrowing toe nail. It should be treated as described under that heading (p. 163).

Subungual epidermoid inclusions

These have been described by Lewin (1969) as bulbous proliferations of the tips of the rete ridges below the nail. They are usually microscopic in size and found only on histological examination of the nail bed. They occur especially with finger clubbing but are also found without this symptom. They may be the result of trauma. Very occasionally they become large enough to cause symptoms and must therefore be considered in the differential diagnosis of nail bed swellings.

Malignant tumours

Epithelioma

Epithelioma of the nail bed is a rare form of malignancy. It is most likely to present as a chronic paronychia with increasing pain (Fig. 11.11), but may present as an outgrowth from below the edge of the nail. It may also begin as a pyogenic granuloma (Driban and Lacagnata, 1975). Biopsy is essential to establish the diagnosis.

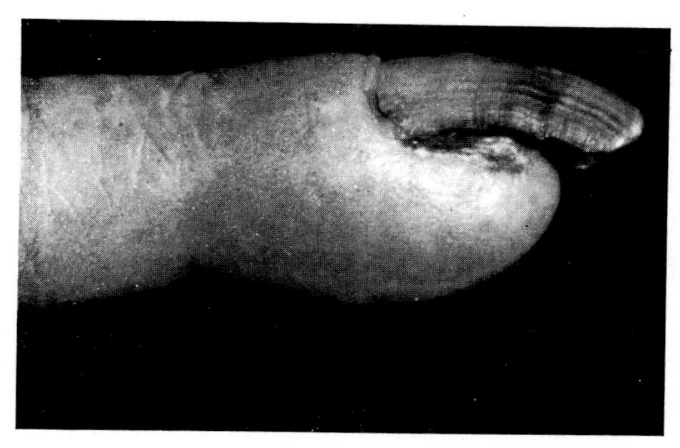

Fig. 11.11 Epithelioma of nail bed presenting as chronic paronychia

Carroll (1976) describes 25 cases, 16 of which were primary and 11 secondary to chronic radiation exposure. The condition had been present for a long time before the diagnosis was made. There were no metastases in these cases. There is a tendency for the distal phalanx to be invaded and it may be destroyed. Treatment should be partial amputation of the digit. Prognosis is good.

Bowen's disease of the nail bed is also rare but should be suspected in any case of gradual destruction of a single nail in the absence of a fungal infection (Fig. 11.12). The condition is liable to progress to an invasive carcinoma. Baran *et al.* (1979) report on five cases and review 20 cases from the literature. The key to the diagnosis lies in the histology. Treatment may be partial amputation of the digit but Moh's chemosurgical technique will give a better cosmetic result (Mikhail, 1974).

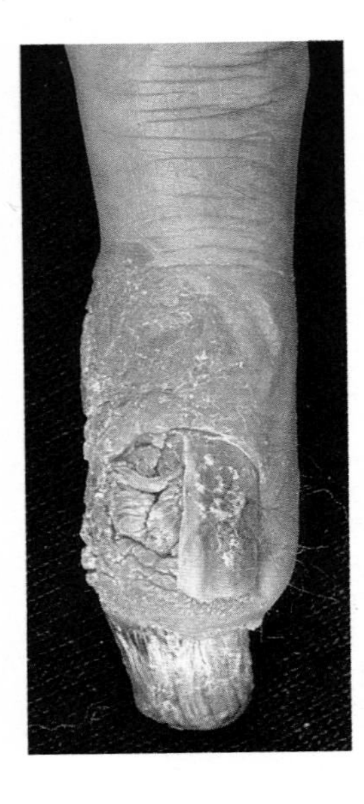

Fig. 11.12 Bowen's disease of nail bed

Defiebre (1978) reports on one case he treated with 5-fluorouracil and a keratolytic ointment.

Secondary carcinoma may occasionally settle in the bone of the distal phalanx giving rise to a painful swelling. X-ray will usually establish the diagnosis, if a primary site is known, but a biopsy may be required.

Malignant melanoma

This also is a rare tumour below the nail but one in which early diagnosis is essential. It may present in various ways, first as a chronic paronychia when the appearance of pigment on the surface of the digit spreading out from below the nail should give rise to suspicion. It may develop from a junctional naevus (p. 176), and in this case the pigment band on the nail will become wider (Fig. 11.13) and granulation tissue may develop at the nail edge. Granulation tissue, resembling a pyogenic granuloma without the added pigment band in the

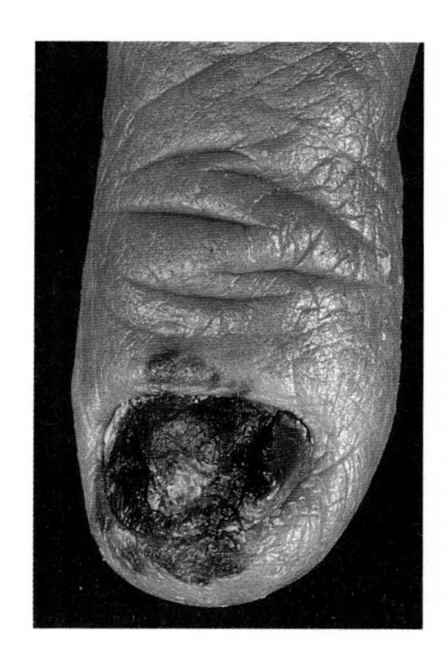

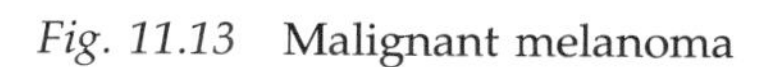
Fig. 11.13 Malignant melanoma

nail, is another presentation. It may also present as a warty thickening of the nail bed with shedding of the nail.

Clark *et al*. (1979) point out that subungual melanomas are usually of a rare type which they call acral lentiginous melanoma (ALM). Overall ALM accounted for only 5.6% of 637 malignant melanomas in the Temple University pigmented lesions study, but 30% of these cases were subungual. Two out of three of these affect the thumb or great toe. The more common superficial spreading and nodular malignant melanomas are very rare below the nails. ALM is a biological form of malignant melanoma with radial and vertical growth phases. The earliest change is pigmentation of the matrix and a halo of pigmentation in the eponychium. This represents Hutchinson's 'melanotic whitlow'. Prognosis is good during the radial growth phase but poor during the vertical growth and change may occur suddenly. Leppard, Sanderson and Baran (1974) point out that unfortunately diagnosis is often much delayed. In any case of doubt a biopsy must be taken. If the diagnosis is confirmed immediate amputation of the digit should be undertaken and the regional nodes should be removed later if necessary. The prognosis is surprisingly good if the diagnosis is made early.

References

Appelberg, D B *et al.* (1979) Subungual osteochondroma. *Arch. Derm.* **115** 472

Arner, O, Lindholm, A and Romanus, R (1956) Mucous cysts of the fingers. *Acta Chir. Scand.* **3** 314

Baran, R, Dupré, A, Sayag, J *et al.* (1979) Bowen disease of the nail apparatus. *Ann. Derm. Venereol.* **106** 227

Bart, R S, Andrade, R, Kopf, A W *et al.* (1968) Acquired digital fibrokeratomas. *Arch. Derm.* **97** 120

Cahn, R L (1977) Acquired periungual fibrokeratoma. *Arch. Derm.* **113** 1564

Carroll, R E (1976) Squamous cell carcinoma of nail bed. *J. Hand Surg.* **1** 92

Clark, W H *et al.* (1979) Acral lentiginous melanoma including melanomas of mucous membranes. In *Human Malignant Melanoma.* (eds Clark, W H, Goldman, I and Mastrangelo, M F). New York: Grune and Stratton

Defiebre, B R Jr (1978) Bowen's disease of the nail bed. *J. Hand Surg.* **3** 184

Driban, N E and Lacagnata, J T (1975) Subungual squamous cell carcinoma. *Derm.* **150** 186

Evison, G (1966) Subungual exostosis. *Brit. J. Radiol.* **39** 451

Halpern, L K and Lane, C W (1953) Treatment of periungual warts. *Missouri Med.* **50** 765

Harvey, K M (1960) Pigmented naevus of nail. *Lancet* **ii** 848

Kikuchi, I, Ishii, Y and Inque, S (1978) Acquired periungual fibroma. *J. Dermatol.* **5** 235

Lamp, J C, Graham, J H, Urbach, F and Burgoon, F Jr (1964) Keratoacanthoma of the subungual region. *J. Bone Jt. Surg.* **46A** 1721

Leppard, B, Sanderson, K V and Baran, R (1974) Subungual malignant melanoma: difficulty in diagnosis. *Brit. Med. J.* **1** 310

Lewin, K (1969) Subungual epidermoid inclusions. *Brit. J. Derm.* **81** 671

Mikhail, G R (1974) Bowen's disease and squamous cell carcinoma of the nail bed. *Arch. Derm.* **110** 267

Pardo-Castello, V and Pardo, O A (1960) *Diseases of the Nails.* 3rd ed., p. 90. Springfield, Illinois: C. C. Thomas

Shelley, W B and Ralston, E I (1964) Paronychia due to echondroma. *Arch. Derm.* **90** 412

Steel, H H (1965) Garlic clove fibroma. *J. Amer. Med. Assoc.* **191** 1082

Stoll, D M and Ackerman, A B (1980) Subungual keratoacanthoma. *Amer. J. Dermatopathol.* **2** 265

Undeutsch, W and Shrieferstein, G (1974) Garlic corm fibroma. *Derm.* **149** 110

Yaffee, M S (1965) Peculiar nail dystrophy caused by an enchondroma. *Arch. Derm.* **91** 361

12

Developmental anomalies

P. D. Samman

Although all rather uncommon developmental anomalies of the nails form an interesting group of disorders, there are a few well-recognised congenital abnormalities and some other conditions which appear to be developmental but where the genetic cause has not yet been firmly established.

Pachyonychia congenita (Figs. 12.1, 12.2)

The term appears first to have been used by Jadassohn and Lewandowski (1906) to describe a case with dystrophic nails, palmar and plantar hyperkeratosis, hyperhidrosis and blistering of the feet during the summer months, excess sweating of the nose and leukokeratosis of the tongue. There have been numerous reports in the literature describing individual cases of families which show several of these features, and others in which the symptomatology is rather different. It is probable that there are a number of different syndromes involved. All are inherited as an autosomal dominant gene but it is uncertain if one or more genes is involved. Kumer and Loos (1935) suggest that there are three main variants. We believe there are four different syndromes as described below.

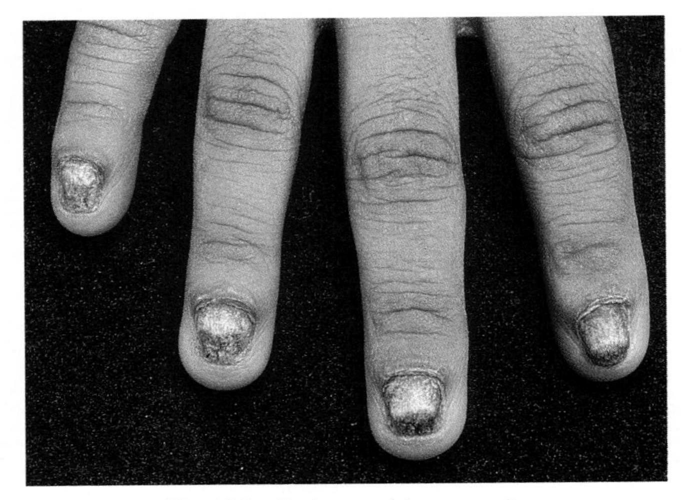

Fig. 12.1 Pachyonychia congenita

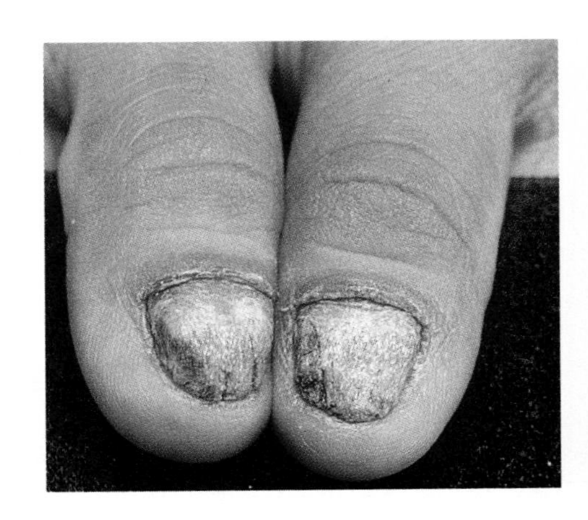

Fig. 12.2 Pachyonychia congenita

Type 1

This is probably the most common and corresponds largely to the original type of Jadassohn and Lewandowski. The nails are usually normal at birth, but within the first year of life, and often in the first few days, they become discoloured and thicken progressively from base to tip so that they appear wedge shaped. This change is seen better on the fingers than the toe nails which are more uniformly thickened. In addition to the nail changes there are characteristically palmar and plantar hyperkeratoses (Fig. 12.3) and warty lesions on knees, elbows, buttocks, legs, ankles and in the popliteal region. Bullae appear on the feet in association with hyperhidrosis and may be crippling. In the mouth, especially on the tongue (Fig. 12.4), there may be dyskeratosis. In some cases corneal dyskeratosis has been described but this has not been seen by the author.

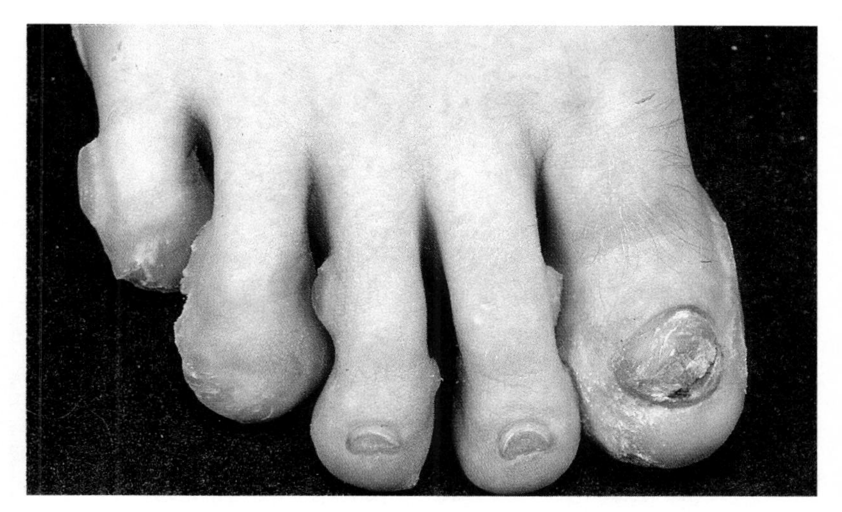

Fig. 12.3 Pachyonychia congenita with hyperkeratotic formation

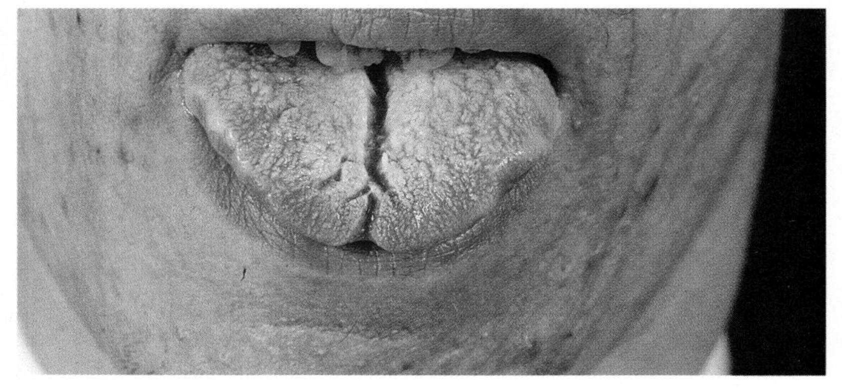

Fig. 12.4 Pachyonychia congenita—tongue showing leukokeratosis

Type 2

In this type the nail thickening is more uniform and some of the nails may be infected with candida (Fig. 12.5). There is also chronic candidiasis in the mouth and this suggests some immune defect. Keratoses are much less severe than in type 1. Patients with chronic oral candidiasis and pachyonychia congenita were shown at the Royal Society of Medicine by Higgs (1973) and Forman and Wells (1975).

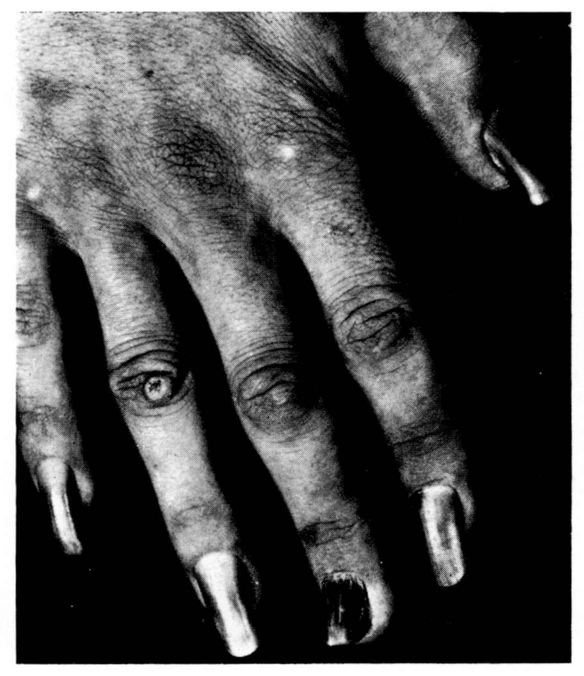

Fig. 12.5 Pachyonychia congenita

Type 3

This is perhaps the most interesting group and is really very different from the other types. Affected children have erupted teeth at birth (Besser, 1971; Murray,1921). Soderquist and Reed (1968) describe such a family where all affected members had two to six teeth at birth. The premature teeth are usually soft and quickly shed but as they normally replace the corresponding milk teeth the children are partially edentulous until the permanent teeth erupt. In this type hyperkeratoses are relatively insignificant and the nail thickening is much less severe than in types 1 and 2. As noted by Shrank (1966) and Soderquist and Reed (1968) adults in these families may have multiple epidermal cysts and there may be other congenital anomalies. Vineyard and Scott (1961) describe the association of sebocystomatosis and pachyonychia congenita and the author has seen such a case in this group. There may also be abnormalities of the hair, which has been variously reported as dry, lustreless and kinky (Soderquist and Reed, 1968), or short and straight and with eyebrows which stand straight out (Boxley, 1971).

Type 4

The characteristic feature in this group is a widespread macular pigmentation affecting especially the neck and axillae. Nail changes and keratoses are of moderate severity.

In addition to the family groups, isolated cases are encountered in which abnormalities are confined to the nails. They should not be called pachyonychia congenita in the absence of other stigmata or a clearcut family history.

Treatment of the whole group is far from satisfactory. The nails should be kept well trimmed and this requires the use of nail clippers. At times the removal of both nail and matrix will be required. Some regrowth from the nail bed should be expected. Hyperkeratotic formations may be helped by the use of salicylic acid or urea ointments. Vitamin A in high dosage has helped some patients, with regard to both keratoses and leukokeratosis. Dupres *et al.* (1981) say that three cases were much helped by the use of the aromatic retinoid RO 109 359.

The nail patella syndrome

This is a curious condition affecting both mesodermal and ectodermal structures. The principal abnormalities consist of nail changes, small or absent patellae, abnormalities of elbow joints, iliac horns and, in a minority of cases, renal changes. It is inherited as an autosomal dominant gene with linkage between the locus controlling the gene and that of the ABO blood groups (Renwick and Lawler, 1955).

The typical case shows nails which are grossly defective, one-third to one-half the normal size and never reaching the fingertip, making it very difficult to pick up small objects (Fig. 12.6). The change is seen more often in women than men. In some cases the entire thumb nail is missing, or it may be represented by a fringe of hard keratin in the nail fold. Although there is scarring it is obvious that the nail bed is present. In the least affected cases only the ulnar half of each thumb nail is missing (Fig. 12.7) while other nails are normal. Levan (1961) described a case of this type and gave a useful bibliography. In every case the thumb nails are most affected and changes, if present in other nails, diminish progressively from index to little finger. A change often seen in the less severely affected nails is a split near the centre dividing the nail, and each half may be spoon-shaped. A V-shaped half moon is also rather characteristic and is the only abnormality seen on some nails (Fig. 12.8).

The abnormality of the patella consists of reduction in size or actual absence. Although the knee appears unstable this abnormality in fact causes very little inconvenience.

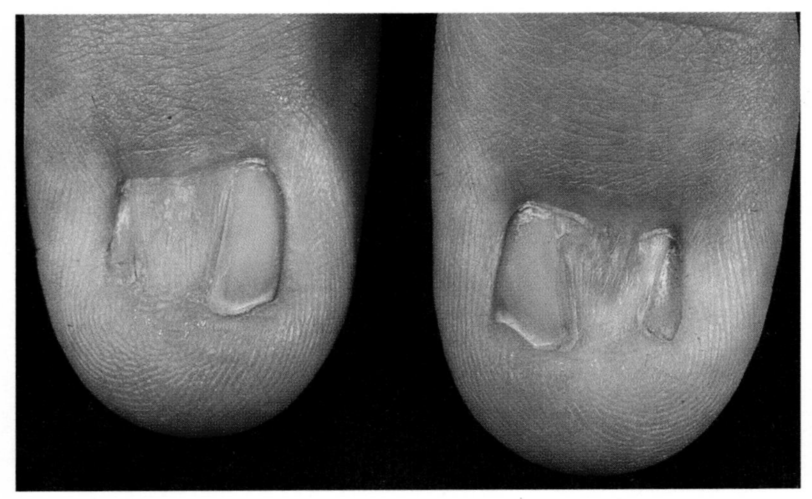

Fig. 12.6 Nail patella syndrome—partial loss of thumb nails

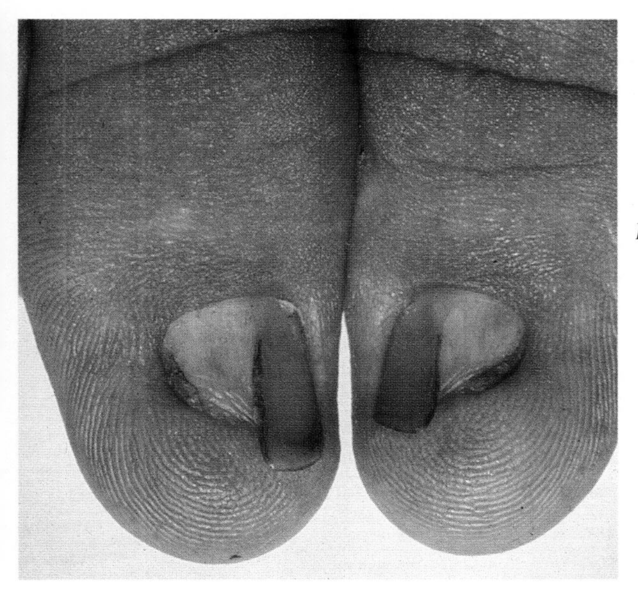

Fig. 12.7 Nail patella syndrome—loss of ulnar half of thumb nails

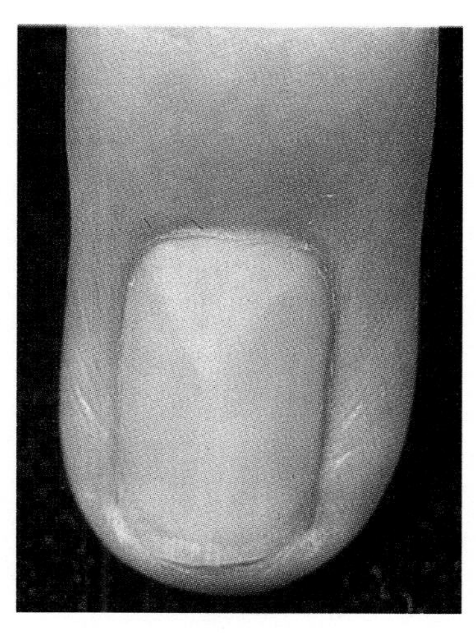

Fig. 12.8 Nail patella syndrome—V-shaped lunula

The elbow joints usually show an obvious deformity. The carrying angle is increased and there is limited supination and incomplete extension of the elbow. In some cases an abnormality is visible only on X-ray. This shows a disorganised joint in which a poorly formed and subluxated head of the radius is articulated with a small underdeveloped capitellum. These changes also cause little inconvenience.

Iliac horns, when large, may be palpated but usually are only seen on X-ray (Fig. 12.9). They arise from the centre of the external aspect of the ilium and project in a posterolateral direction.

Agarwal *et al.* (1974) described cases in an Indian family. The father of the propositors had other abnormalities, namely deformity of the fingers of the left hand and flexion deformities of the proximal interphalangeal joints of the right hand. Pierard and de la Brassinne (1974) describe cases of three patients in five generations who also suffered from spina bifida.

The renal changes clinically are those of chronic glomerulonephritis with persistent albuminuria and casts of all types, and occasional red blood cells in the urine. Renal function may be diminished (Hawkins and Smith, 1950). Although the other changes are usually present in all affected individuals the renal changes are inconstant and are the only serious

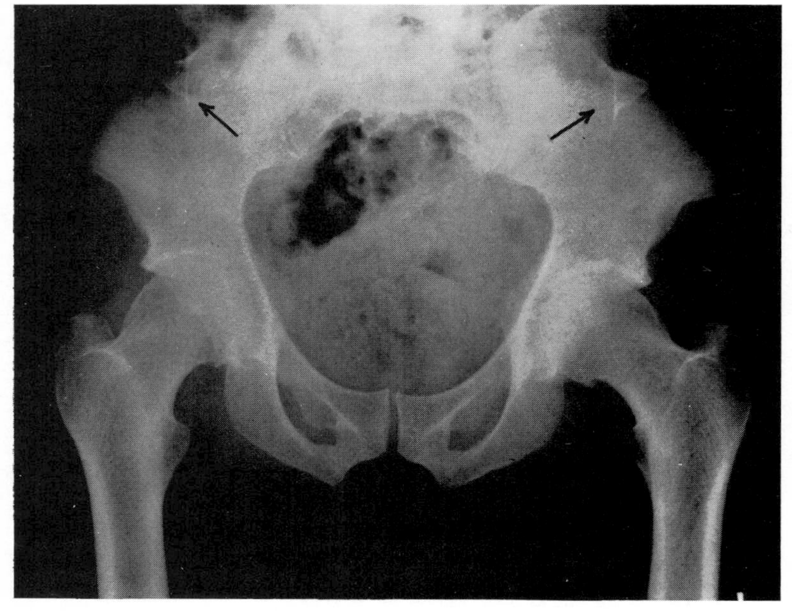

Fig. 12.9 Nail patella syndrome—X-ray pelvis showing iliac spines (arrowed)

feature of the syndrome. Goodman and Cuppage (1967) and Ben-Basset, Cohen and Rosenfeld (1971) have examined the kidney under the electronmicroscope and showed that the changes include thickening and wrinkling of the glomerular basement membrane.

Anonychia

Apart from the nail patella syndrome anonychia (absence of the nail from birth) is encountered very rarely. Littman and Levin (1964) described a girl with seven nails missing; her brother was similarly affected. They considered the condition to be an autosomal recessive genetic defect. In anonychia with ectrodactyly (Lees *et al.*, 1957) several nails may be missing and there are often bizarre associated defects of the digits. This is an autosomal dominant condition. Feinmesser and Zelig (1961) described two children of a sibship of five with rudimentary nails and an associated congenital deafness. Verbov (1975) described a case with anonychia, bizarre flexural pigmentation, hypohidrosis and dry palmar and plantar skin which partly destroyed the normal skin markings. Other members of the family were similarly affected with autosomal dominant inheritance.

Bart (1971) gives details of a family showing a unique combination of localised absence of the skin, blistering of skin and mucous membranes and nail abnormalities. The nail deformities consist of congenital absence, or subsequent loss and other changes. He refers to an earlier description of the family in which the blistering was likened to epidermolysis bullosa. The condition showed an autosomal dominant mode of inheritance.

Congenital ectodermal defect

There are a number of different syndromes described under this heading, the main division being into anhidrotic and hidrotic types. Ellis and Dawber (1980) remind us that there are more than two types and that teeth may be involved as well as nails and hair.

In the usual anhidrotic type nail changes are an insignificant feature but they may be thin, brittle and ridged.

Hidrotic type

This condition is inherited as an autosomal dominant and many of the recorded cases can be traced to a small region in France. Clouston (1929) described a large number of cases from the French-speaking part of Canada. In every case the nails were involved, and the hair in 50% of cases. Rajagopalan and Tay (1977) report on a large Chinese pedigree.

Various nail changes have been described. The most characteristic seen in several patients by the author is a nail which grows slowly and never reaches the fingertip. Surrounding the nail, and on the fingertip including the nail bed left exposed by the failure of the nail to reach the tip, is a curious mammilation (Figs. 12.10, 12.11), seen on all fingers. Onycholysis is the principal feature in other cases and this may be accompanied by subungual sepsis and malodour. Toe nails are more often

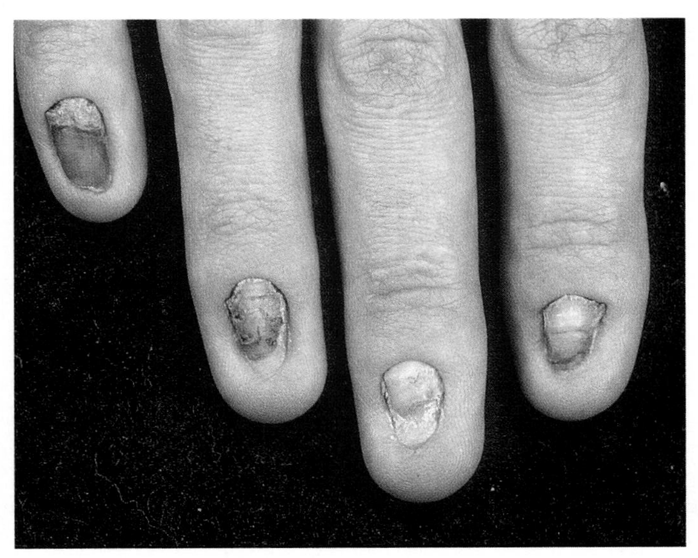

Fig. 12.10 Congenital ectodermal defect (hidrotic type)—fingers showing failure of nails to grow to full length and mammilation of fingertips

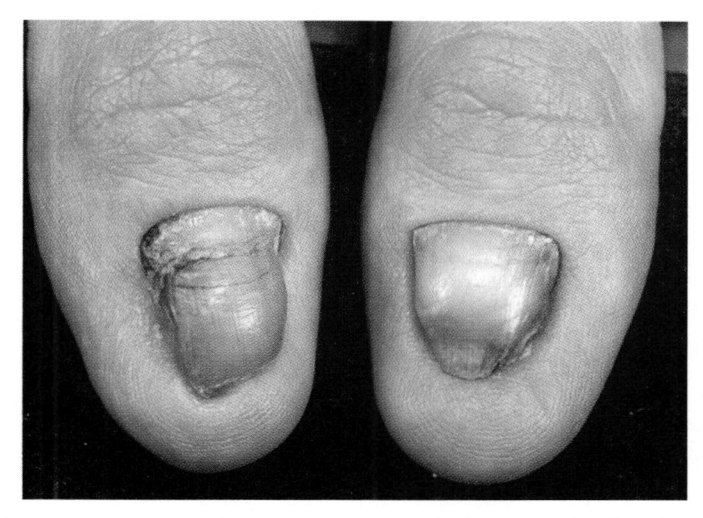

Fig. 12.11 Congenital ectodermal defect (hidrotic type)—thumb nails showing thickening and discoloration

thickened and the mammilation is less obvious. Pachyonychial changes are sometimes present. Other nail changes have been described, but it is not clear from the literature that they refer to the hidrotic type, and there is undoubted confusion between this condition and the nail patella syndrome.

Alopecia (Fig. 12.12) seen in half the cases may involve the scalp alone or be universal. There are often hyperkeratotic formations on the soles and elsewhere.

Dyskeratosis congenita

Various nail abnormalities have been recorded in this very rare disorder (Cole, Rauskolb and Toomey, 1930).

Racket nail

This is in fact a congenital abnormality of the thumb (*le pouce en raquette*) with the nail conforming to the altered shape of the thumb. It is very much more common than the other conditions described here. It is inherited as an autosomal dominant

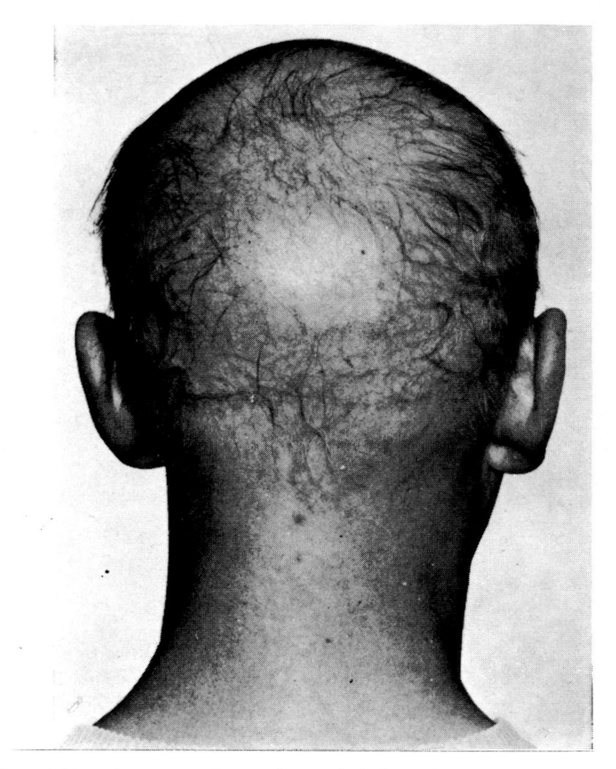

Fig. 12.12 Congenital ectodermal defect (hidrotic type)—alopecia

but is rather more common in women than men—Basset (1962) says twice as common, and Ronchese (1973) three times as common. It may affect one or both thumbs. The distal phalanx is shorter and wider than usual and the nail is also short and wide and the lateral curvature is lost (Fig. 12.13). Of 63 cases investigated by Ronchese (1951) 31 gave a family history.

Basset (1962) distinguished this from two similar conditions. In one the racket shape affects all fingers and in the other the thumb nails are short but without the corresponding shortening of the distal phalanges.

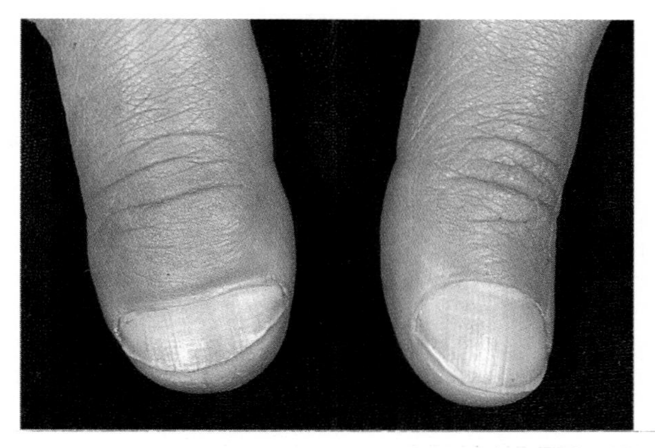

Fig. 12.13 Nail *en raquette*

Supernumerary digits

These are usually provided with a normal nail but when rudimentary there may either be no sign of the nail or nail matrix or the tip is provided with a vestigial nail (Fig. 12.14).

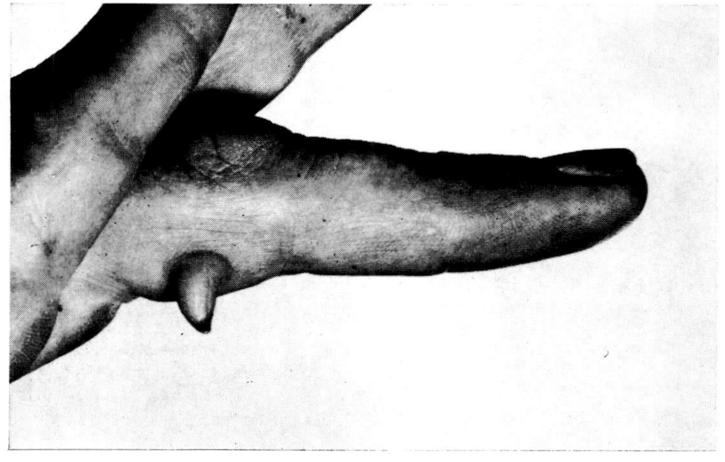

Fig. 12.14 Rudimentary supernumerary digit with vestigial nail

Congenital onychodysplasia of the index fingers (COIF)

There have been a number of papers describing this condition (Kikuchi, Horikawa and Amano, 1974; Baran 1980; Baran and Stroud 1984), and the name used here is not universally accepted because not every case is confined to the index fingers. There is a genetic factor in some cases.

The index finger nails of affected cases are absent, small or multiple, and probably the commonest change is the presence of two small nails on one finger, the nail on the radial side of the digit being the smaller (Fig. 12.15). A possible explanation for this is that the condition is due to ischaemia in fetal life and the digital vessel on the radial side is smaller than that on the ulnar side and more likely to become occluded. The condition may affect one or both index fingers.

Most of the early cases were reported from Japan, but a few have since been reported from other parts of the world including the United Kingdom (Samman, 1983).

In addition to the nail changes there may be other abnormalities, mainly of the hands. X-rays may show hypoplasia and narrowing of the distal third of the distal phalanx and bifurcation at the tip of the distal phalanx.

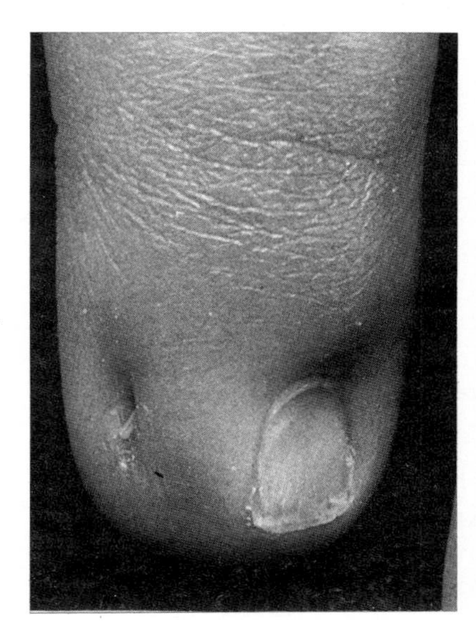

Fig. 12.15 Congenital onychodysplasia of the index finger

Leukonychia totalis

This is a rare developmental abnormality inherited as an autosomal dominant. The entire nail plate is white, the whiteness being due to changes in the nail plate itself. The material of the nail is poor and it may become brittle, broken and discoloured distally (Fig. 12.16). In many cases multiple epidermal cysts are also present. Bushkell and Jensen (1975) describe an example spreading over four generations where renal calculi were also present.

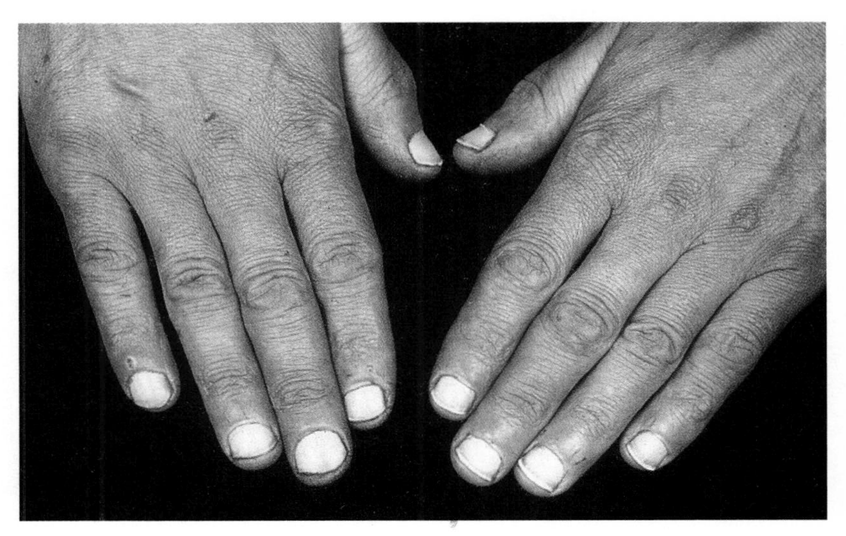

Fig. 12.16 Leukonychia totalis

Periodic shedding

This is another rare developmental abnormality which is inherited as an autosomal dominant. One or more nails is repeatedly shed and replaced. The new nail may be imperfect and this leads to considerable deformities (Fig. 12.17). The nails on various digits are shed independently so that there is seldom more than one missing at a time.

The true congenital condition must be distinguished from shedding due to other causes and in particular from trauma due to footwear.

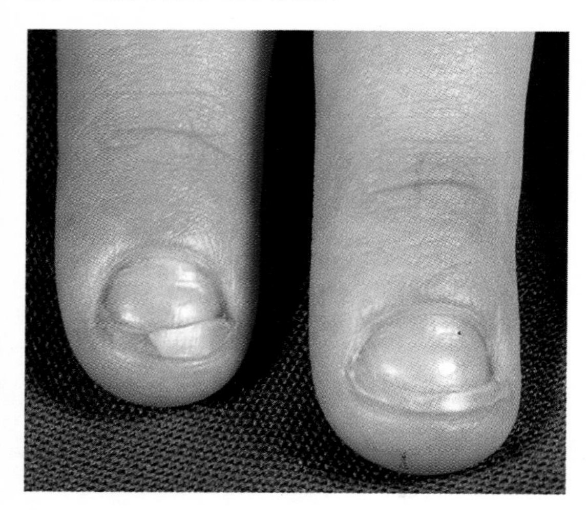

Fig. 12.17 Periodic shedding

A very curious case of nail shedding was described by Frank and Sanford (1891), whose patient shed his whole epidermis including all nails on the same day every year for 45 years. Other cases of a similar nature have been recorded.

Hereditary koilonychia has been described on p. 111, and onycholysis on p. 25. A developmental form described as hereditary partial onycholysis has been described by Schulze (1966). Sparrow, Samman and Wells (1976) recorded details of a family showing hyperpigmentation, hypohidrosis, nail dystrophy, hypoplasia of dermatoglyphics and a number of other abnormalities. The main nail change was extensive onycholysis.

Conditions of unknown aetiology

Trachyonychia (rough nails)

Alkiewicz (1950) and Achten and Wanet-Rouard (1974) use the term *trachyonychie* to describe rough nails. Baran and Dupré (1977) elaborate and say that rough nails are suggestive of some cases of alopecia areata and use the term 'vertical striated sandpaper nails' to describe these cases. When the vertical striations do not cover the full expanse of the nail plates the condition, they say, may be due to lichen planus or psoriasis.

The author has seen many cases of rough nails which are very difficult to place aetiologically and roughly divides them into the following groups (Samman, 1979):

(1) Universal pitting with variants excess ridging and rippling.
(2) Excess ridging (not a manifestation of universal pitting) and sometimes called '20-nail dystrophy'.
(3) Alopecia areata.
(4) Severe nail dystrophy.

Regular pitting

Many cases of uniform pitting of the nails can be attributed to psoriasis (Klingmüller and Reh, 1955) or to alopecia areata (Stühmer, 1957) but when these conditions have been excluded, by personal and family history and by examination, some unexplained cases remain (Fig. 12.18). Several examples have been seen in more than one member of a

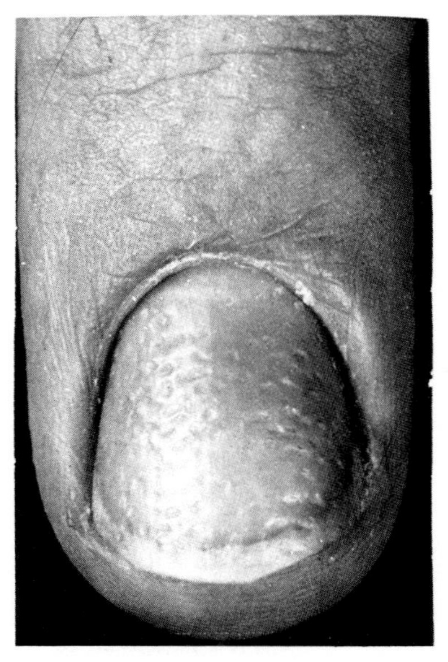

Fig. 12.18 Regular pitting—cause unknown

family, so some genetic basis is probable. The pits usually appear early in life but may become manifest years later. One or many nails are affected. The patient can observe the change starting as pits which become visible in the half moon area and progress forwards to involve the whole nail. Mottling in the half moon is sometimes present. The condition may gradually clear spontaneously but more often it is permanent. It is apparent that there is an intermittent defect of parts of the matrix, the cause of which is as yet unknown.

Excess ridging and rippling

These two conditions appear at times to be variants of uniform pitting and patients have been seen where all three abnormalities were present at the same time on different digits (Fig. 12.19). The manner in which regular pitting could produce these changes is shown in Fig. 12.20. As the aetiology is obscure it is possible that there is more than one cause and not every case will be genetically determined. Rippling gives a

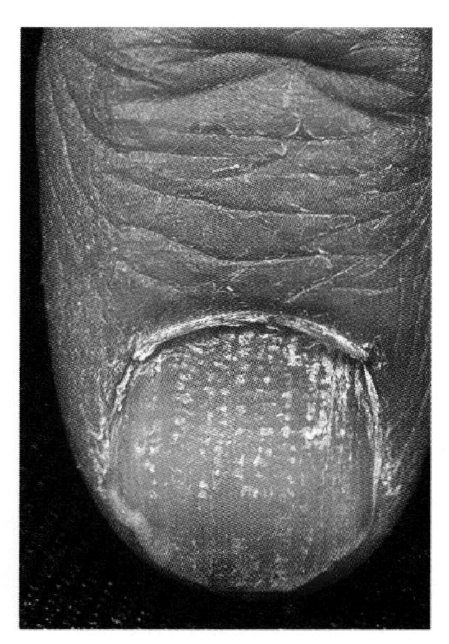

Fig. 12.19 Ridging of finger nail

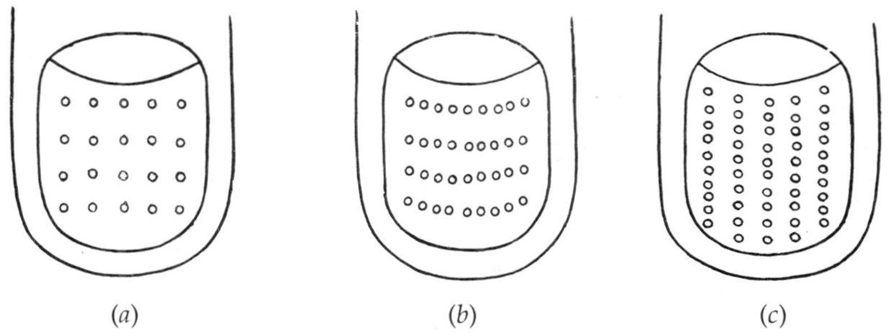

Fig. 12.20 Diagrams to show how (a) regular pitting could be converted to (b) rippling or (c) ridging

very characteristic picture similar to the ripples on the sand of the sea shore after the tide has gone out (Fig. 12.21).

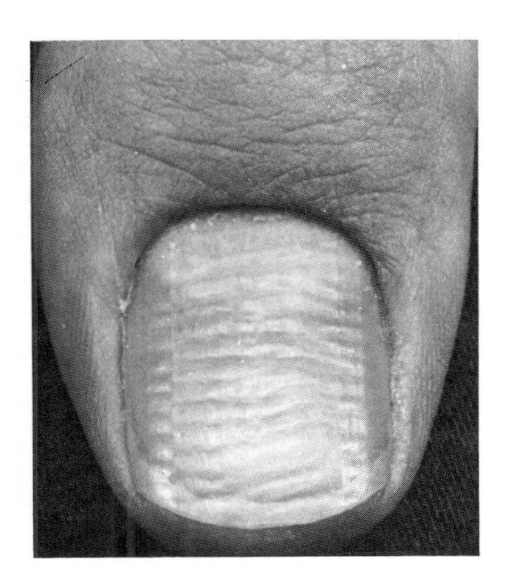

Fig. 12.21 Rippling

Twenty-nail dystrophy of childhood

Hazelrigg, Duncan and Jarratt (1977) give this name to a condition which was described in earlier editions of this book under the heading of excess ridging. Excess ridging appears to be the primary defect and in this case is not due to multiple pits running together. The child is born with normal nails but after a few months or years all nails become excessively ridged (Fig. 12.22). The ridging starts at the cuticle and progresses to the tip. There are so many lines close together that the nail loses its lustre and becomes opalescent; the end result is a

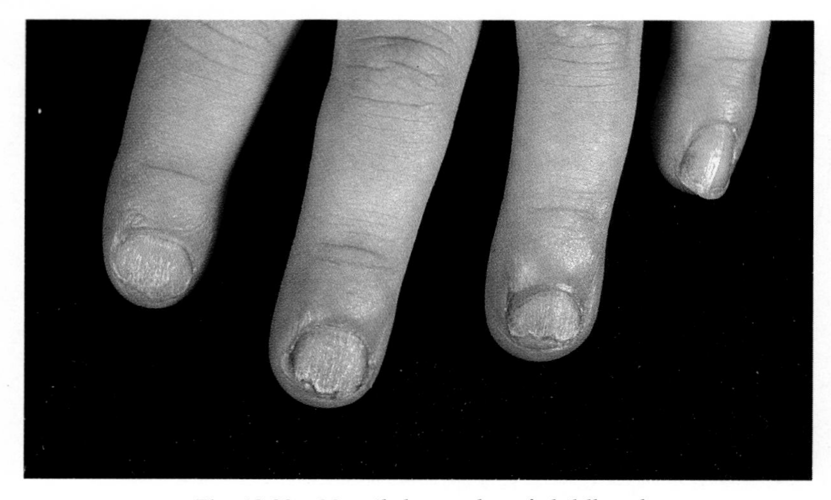

Fig. 12.22 20-nail dystrophy of childhood

rather ugly nail (Fig. 12.23). There are no related skin or hair abnormalities. In the majority of cases there is no family history of a similar disorder but the author has seen two cases in one family, both girls. The dystrophy is at its worst in the early stage and gradually decreases with age. As it is seldom encountered in adults it seems probable that eventually it clears entirely. Treatment has little effect on progress, but the use of nail lacquer hides the defect.

Severe nail dystrophy

This is another condition usually seen in childhood and affecting many nails. It has to be distinguished from psoriasis and alopecia areata affecting the nails and this may not be easy. The nails are affected in a variety of ways and all types of change may occur at the same time, one nail showing one form while others show another. Often some nails are completely spared. Most nails are soft, slightly discoloured, opalescent and lack lustre (Figs. 12.24, 12.25). Some are thicker than normal but some are thin. Pitting or ridging may be present but this is not a prominent feature. Some nails, especially thumb or great toe nails, show marked koilonychia. Although most cases are seen in young children and, as in the 20-nail dystrophy, there is a gradual improvement with

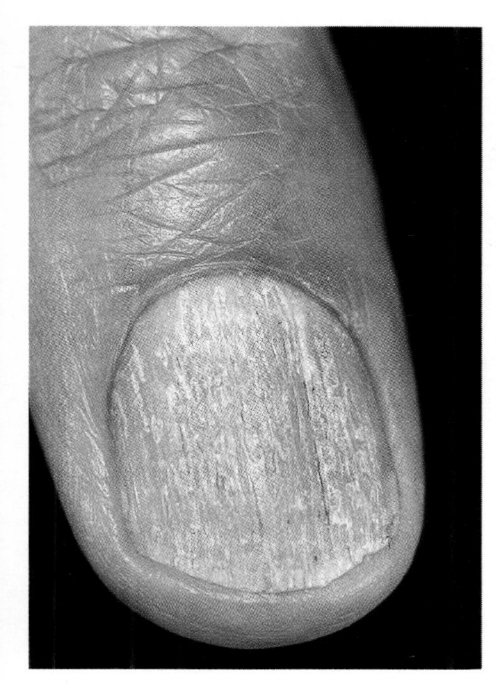

Fig. 12.23 Nail with excess ridging

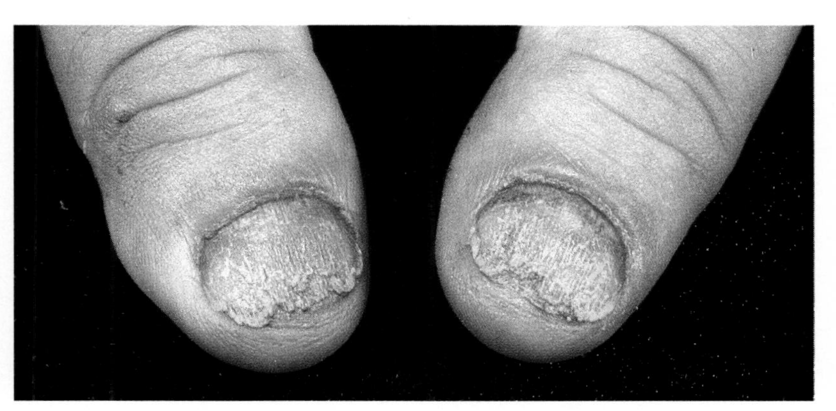

Fig. 12.24 Severe nail dystrophy

age, a few cases have been found in adults. Injections of triamcinolone have improved the adult cases but have not been used in young children. The author usually recommends the use of a relatively mild topical steroid but it is uncertain whether this treatment really helps.

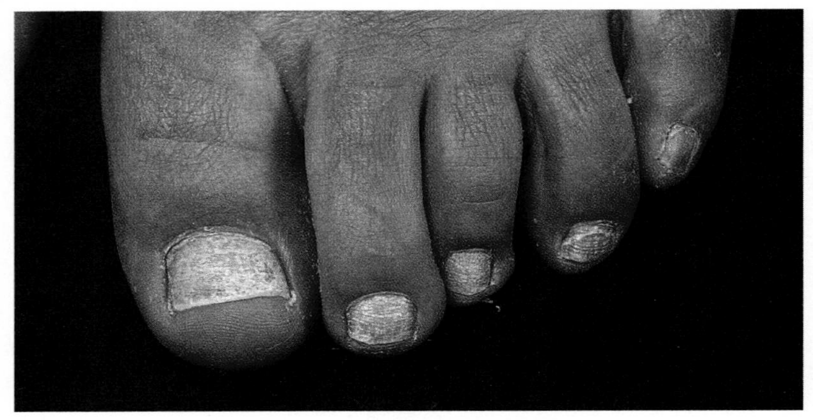

Fig. 12.25 Severe nail dystrophy

The term trachyonychia covers all these conditions but it must be realised that it is a symptom and not a specific disease.

Congenital malalignment of the big toe nail

Samman (1978) was the first to describe this condition under the name 'Great toe nail dystrophy'. Baran, Bureau and Sayag (1979) soon followed using the more suitable name given here. It is a condition confined to one or both great toe nails. The nail changes are present at birth. The nail is dark coloured, slightly pointed but shorter than a normal nail (Fig. 12.26). Cross-ridges may develop on its surface and a large portion of the nail may be shed from time to time. In a number of cases the condition has been entirely symptomless except for the disfigurement, but, in one child, after shedding of part of the nail, ingrowth into the nail bed occurred on regrowth so that the nail had to be removed surgically. Baran, Bureau and Sayag (1979) maintain that the defect can be corrected by a surgical procedure to the matrix in which the whole nail apparatus is realigned. They say that early recognition and surgery will prevent trouble in later life (see also p. 217).

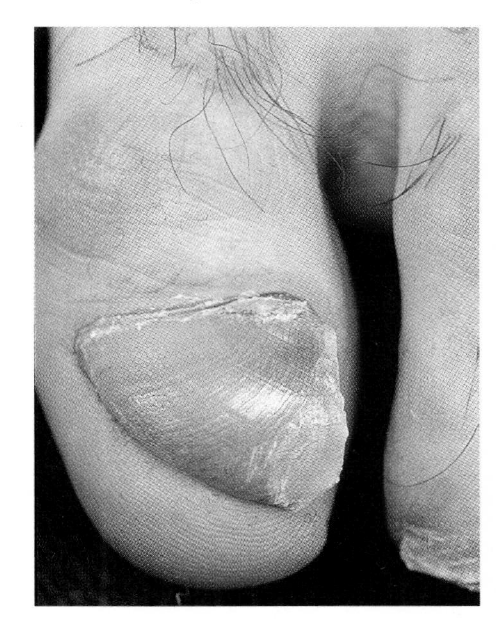

Fig. 12.26 Congenital malalignment

Dawson (1979) describes two families in which a nail dystrophy principally affecting the great toe nails gave an appearance similar to malalignment. The author has also seen congenital malalignment of the second toe nail (Fig. 12.27).

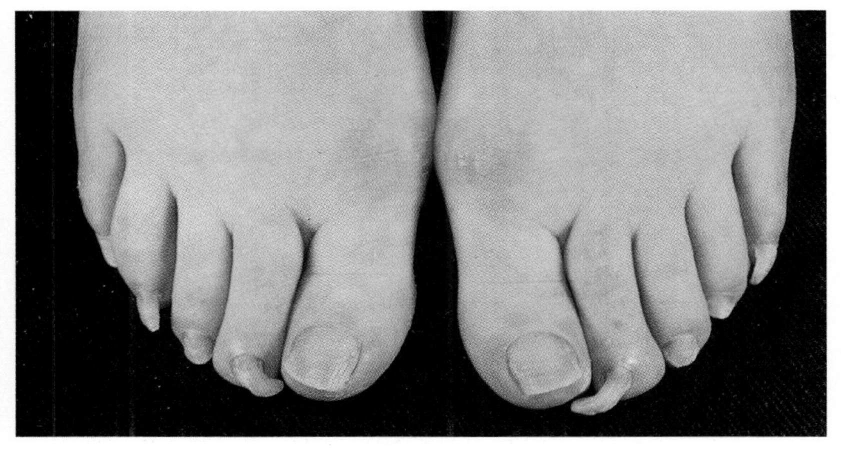

Fig. 12.27 Congenital malalignment of the second toe nail

Macronychia and micronychia

These are nails which are larger (macro) or smaller (micro) (Fig. 12.28) than normal but in all other respects are quite normal. The condition may affect one or more nails and be unilateral or bilateral.

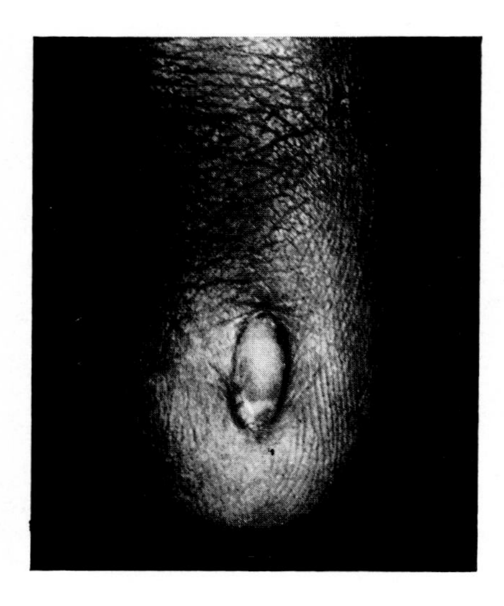

Fig. 12.28 Micronychia

Claw-like little toe nails

These are not uncommon. One or both little toe nails are rounded like a claw, and the condition is often associated with hyperkeratotic formations on the feet or elsewhere. Much less often other toe nails show this change.

References

Achten, G and Wanet-Rouard, J (1974) Atrophie unguale et trachyonchie. *Arch. Belges Derm.* **30** 201

Agarwal, V K *et al.* (1974) An Indian family with the nail patella syndrome. *Ind. J. Pediat.* **41** 364

Alkiewicz, J (1950) Trachyonychie. *Ann. Derm. Syph.* **10** 136

Baran, R (1980) Syndrome d'Iso et Kikuchi. *Ann. Derm. Véner.* **107** 431

Baran, R and Dupré, A (1977) Vertical striated sandpaper nails (letter). *Arch. Derm.* **113** 1613

Baran, R, Bureau, H and Sayag, J (1979) Congenital malalignment of the big toe nail. *Clin. Exp. Derm.* **4** 359

Baran, R and Stroud, J D (1984) Congenital onychodysplasia of the index fingers. *Arch. Derm.* **120** 243

Bart, B J (1971) Congenital localised absence of skin, blistering and nail abnormalities, a new syndrome. *Birth defects: original article series* **7** 118

Basset, M R H (1962) Trois formes génotypiques d'ongles courts: le pouce en raquette, les doigts en raquette, les ongles courts simples. *Bull. Soc. Fr. Derm. Syph.* **69** 15

Ben-Basset, M, Cohen, L and Rosenfeld, J (1971) The glomerular basement membrane in the nail patella syndrome. *Arch. Path.* **92** 350

Besser, F S (1971) Pachyonychia congenita with epidermal cysts and teeth at birth: 4th generation. *Brit. J. Derm.* **84** 95

Boxley, J D (1971) Pachyonychia congenita and multiple epidermal haematomata. *Brit. J. Derm.* **85** 298

Bushkell, L L and Jensen, G (1975) Leukonychia totalis, multiple sebaceous cysts and renal circuit. A syndrome. *Birth Defects: original article series* **11** 19

Clouston, H R (1929) A hereditary ectodermal dystrophy. *Can. Med. Assoc. J.* **21** 18

Cole, H N, Rauskolb, J E and Toomey, J (1930) Dyskeratosis congenita with pigmentation, dystrophia unguis and leukokeratosis oris. *Arch. Derm.* **21** 71

Dawson, J A J (1979) An inherited nail dystrophy principally affecting the great toe nails. *Clin. Exp. Derm.* **4** 309

Dupres, A *et al.* (1981) Familial pachyonychia. *Ann. Derm Venereol. (Paris)* **108** 145

Ellis, J and Dawber, R P R (1980) Ectodermal dysplasia syndrome, a family study. *Clin. Exp. Derm.* **5** 295

Feinmesser, M and Zelig, S (1961) Congenital deafness associated with onychodystrophy. *Arch. Otolar.* **74** 507

Forman, L and Wells, R S (1975) Pachyonychia congenita and chronic candidiasis of the mouth in the father and two children. *Proc. Roy. Soc. Med.* **68** 762

Frank, J and Sanford, W C (1891) A remarkable case of skin disease. *Amer. J. Med. Sci.* **102** 164

Goodman, R M and Cuppage, F E (1967) The nail patella syndrome. Clinical findings and ultrastructural observations in the kidney. *Arch. Intern. Med.* **120** 68

Hawkins, C F and Smith, O E (1950) Renal dysplasia in a family with multiple hereditary abnormalities including iliac horns. *Lancet* **i** 803

Hazelrigg, D E, Duncan, C and Jarratt, M (1977) Twenty nail dystrophy of childhood. *Arch. Derm.* **113** 75

Higgs, J M (1973) Pachyonychia congenita and chronic oral candidiasis. *Proc. Roy. Soc. Med.* **66** 628

Jadassohn von, J and Lewandowski, F (1906) Pachyonychia congenita. Keratosis disseminata circumscripta tylomata et keratosis linguae. *Ikonographia Derm.*

Kikuchi, I, Horikawa, S and Amano, S (1974) Congenital onychodysplasia of the index finger. *Arch. Derm.* **110** 743

Klingmüller, G and Reh, E (1955) Nagelbrübchen und deren familiäre Haüfungen bei der Alopecia areata. *Arch. Klin. Exp. Derm.* **201** 574

Kumer, L and Loos, H O (1955) Uber pachyonychia congenita (typus Riehl). *Wein. Klin. Washa.* **6** 174

Lees, D H, Lawler, S D, Renwick, J H and Thoday, J M (1957) Anonychia with ectrodactyly: clinical and linkage data. *Ann. Hum. Genet.* **22** 69

Levan, N E (1961) Congenital defect of thumb nails. *Arch. Derm.* **83** 938

Littman, A and Levin, S (1964) Anonychia as a recessive autosomal trait in man. *J. Invest. Derm.* **42** 177

Murray, F A (1921) Congenital anomalies of the nails. Four cases of hereditary hypertrophy of the nail-bed associated with a history of erupted teeth at birth. *Brit. J. Derm.* **33** 409

Pierard, R P and de la Brassinne, M (1974) Nail patella syndrome. *Arch. Belges Derm.* **30** 259

Rajagopalan, K and Tay, C H (1977) Hidrotic ectodermal dysplasia. Study of a large Chinese pedigree. *Arch. Derm.* **113** 481

Renwick, J H and Lawler, S D (1955) Genetical linkage between the A B O and nail patella loci. *Ann. Hum. Genet. (Lond.)* **19** 312

Ronchese, F (1951) Peculiar nail anomalies. *Arch. Derm.* **63** 565

Ronchese, F (1973) The racket thumb-nail. *Dermatologica* **146** 199

Samman, P D (1978) Great toe nail dystrophy. *Clin. Exp. Derm.* **3** 81

Samman, P D (1979) Trachyonychia (rough nails). *Brit. J. Derm.* **101** 701

Samman, P D (1983) Congenital onychodysplasia of the index fingers. *Clin. Exp. Derm.* **8** 563

Schulze, H D (1966) Hereditäre onycholysis partialis mit Skleronychie. *Derm. Washa.* **152** 766

Shrank, A B (1966) Pachyonychia congenita (case report). *Proc. Roy. Soc. Med.* **59** 975

Soderquist, N A and Reed, W B (1968) Pachyonychia congenita with epidermal cysts and other congenital dyskeratoses. *Arch. Derm.* **97** 31

Sparrow, G P, Samman, P D and Wells, R S (1976) Hyperpigmentation and hypohidrosis. *Clin. Exp. Derm.* **1** 127

Stühmer, A (1957) Rhythmen im biologischen Gescheben bei gesunden und kranken Nägeln. *Arch. Klin. Exp. Derm.* **204** 1

Verbov, J (1975) Anonychia with bizarre flexural pigmentation—an autosomal dominant dermatosis. *Brit. J. Derm.* **92** 469

Vineyard, W R and Scott, R A (1961) Steatocystoma multiplex with pachyonychia congenita. *Arch. Derm.* **84** 824

13

Nail surgery

R. P. R. Dawber and R. Baran

In general, dermatologists seem averse to undertaking nail surgical procedures. This frequently applies even to clinicians who are competent and well qualified to carry out skin surgery. It is surprising that this is so in view of the good blood supply, and the well-recognised rapid healing of the nail apparatus after injury. The major limiting factors appear to be the lack of experienced nail surgeons to act as trainers, and the fact that the consequences of poor surgical technique are great because of the importance of a normal nail to the efficient functioning of each digit.

In this chapter particular attention is given to those techniques that are within the compass of dermatology department facilities for the diagnosis and treatment of common lesions and dermatoses (Bureau, Baran and Haneke, 1984).

The major objectives in carrying out nail surgery are (1) to obtain diagnostic, therapeutic or prognostic information by nail biopsy; (2) to treat nail tumours; (3) to relieve pain; (4) to treat infections; and (5) to repair or correct congenital and traumatic deformities.

To obtain the best functional and cosmetic results from nail surgery, careful attention should be given to maintaining the relationship of the component parts of the nail apparatus to each other where possible.

Examination of the patient

Careful history-taking is essential prior to surgery to exclude high-risk patients, for example those with peripheral vascular disease, diabetes, blood dyscrasias and connective tissue diseases. Drugs being taken for other reasons may interfere with the procedure—for example, aspirin can prolong bleeding, phenothiazines or monoamine oxidase inhibitors (MAOIs) can interfere with anaesthesia, and oral and topical steroids can delay healing. A history of allergy to local anaesthetics or preservatives should be sought.

Preoperative preparation

Minimising the risk of infection is important. This can be achieved by the use of preoperative antiseptic methods such as scrubbing the area with providine-iodine or chlorhexidine and then applying the equivalent tincture or presurgery preparation.

Anaesthesia

There are many alternative agents available and the main consideration for the operator is to be familiar with the agent chosen with regard to its speed of onset, duration of action and potency. The amide group have a lower allergy potential than the esters. Lignocaine (for example Xylocaine) is the most widely used local anaesthetic, acting more rapidly (within minutes) and being more stable than other agents; 1% is the strength most frequently used, and it acts for approximately 2 hours. Preparations containing epinephrine should not be used in nail surgery since digital gangrene may develop if vasospasm is prolonged.

Nail surgery is usually carried out under proximal digital ('ring'-block') anaesthesia; more distal injections should never be used in the presence of infection—if the latter is severe, nerve trunk anaesthesia of the median, radial or ulnar nerve at the wrist may be more appropriate. A tourniquet to the digit to provide a bloodless field may be necessary for nail surgery procedures; it can be left *in situ* for up to 15 minutes.

Nail biopsy

Most biopsy techniques in the nail area are quick, simple to carry out and cause no greater functional impairment or scarring than any other skin biopsy technique (Bureau, Baran and Haneke, 1984). Zaias (1967) pioneered the use of histological examination for nail pathology. The best cytological results are obtained if the tissue is embedded in Araldite and cut with an ultramicrotome.

The actual technique used depends on the site to be biopsied and the information required. Fig. 13.1 shows the commonest biopsy sites. The punch biopsy technique may be used on any part of the nail apparatus, but it is limited by the small amount of normal tissue obtained. The most radical technique, the longitudinal biopsy of Zaias (1967) gives information regarding every component of the nail apparatus (Fig. 13.2). The wedge of tissue removed should not exceed 3 mm in width or a permanent defect may occur; central biopsies may cause a distal split and consequently lateral sections should be obtained where possible to minimise this defect.

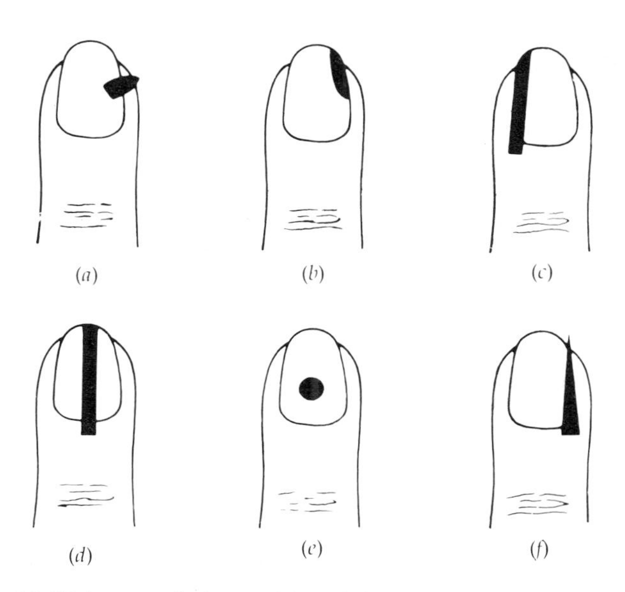

Fig. 13.1 Nail biopsy techniques; (*a*) and (*b*) are often used for histological or mycological examination (Achten); (*c*), (*f*)—personal techniques; (*d*)—longitudinal biopsy (Zaias); (*e*)—punch biopsy

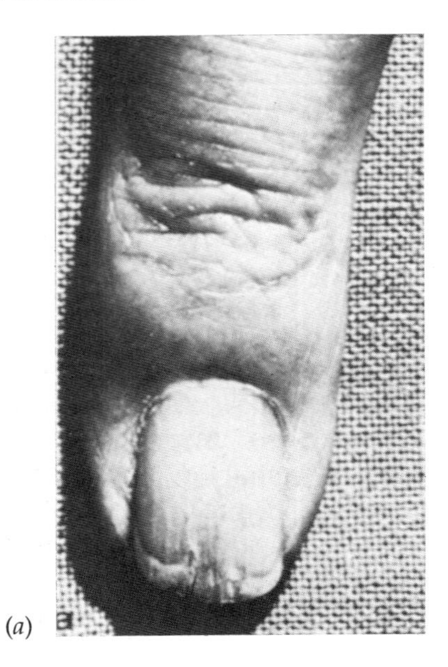

(*a*)

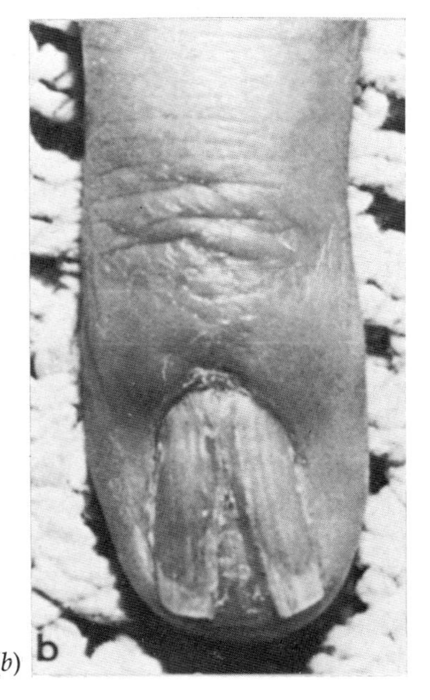

(*b*)

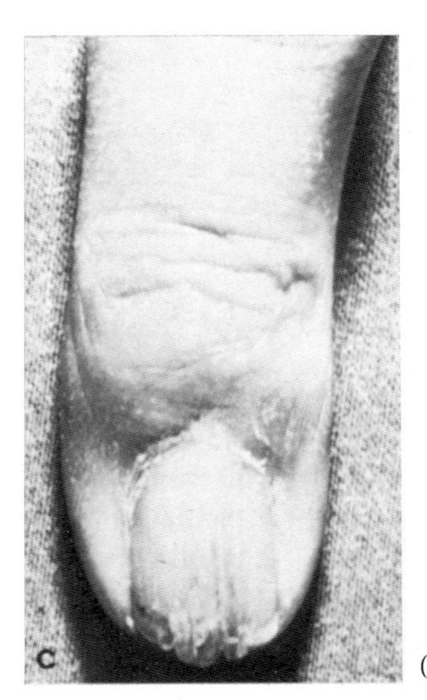

(*c*)

Fig. 13.2 Longitudinal biopsy (Zaias); (*a*) before (*b*) 1 month and (*c*) 6 months after the procedure

superficial sampling may lead to inadequate intermediate matrix and nail bed dermis in the specimen; there being no subcutaneous fat, the dermal connective tissue bonds directly to periosteum.

Some biopsy methods have evolved to resolve specific diagnostic problems. In attempting to differentiate between psoriasis and primary fungal disease when the nail and nail bed are grossly thickened and fungal microscopy and culture are negative, it is useful to remove a wedge of thickened subungual keratin and process it using routine histological methods with PAS or silver methenamine staining to define fungal invasion; if psoriasis is the diagnosis, parakeratosis and polymorph debris will be seen microscopically (Scher and Ackerman, 1980). In proximal subungual onychomycosis a small punch biopsy may be required to obtain the necessary affected tissue for fungal microscopy and culture. If a longitudinal pigmented band develops and malignant melanoma is possibly the cause, a punch biopsy technique can be used. The proximal nail fold is reflected off the nail plate and a specimen taken from the proximal end of the pigmented streak, by a punch biopsy taken through the nail plate which is soft in this region, or a punch biopsy or transverse wedge biopsy of the same site after removing the proximal half of the nail plate.

Proximal nail fold (PNF) biopsy has been recommended for the study of connective tissue diseases; a crescent-shaped 'slice' of the full thickness of the proximal nail fold is removed with a sharp blade such as a single-edged razor blade. The tissue obtained enables useful light-microscopic, immunoscopic and electronmicroscopic studies to be carried out. Since the matrix is not damaged, no nail dystrophy occurs.

Nail avulsion

This process is most commonly carried out by a distal method under proximal digital anaesthesia. Straight haemostatis forceps are used; adjacent to the lateral nail fold, one jaw is pushed proximally, deep to the nail plate, until it reaches the nail matrix area. Prior to this the proximal nail fold is reflected off the nail after two incisions have been made through it in line with the lateral nail grooves. The forceps jaws are then closed, the nail plate between them, and the instrument rotated in a manner analogous to opening a sardine can. Little force is necessary to remove the nail by this method.

Since in the matrix area the nail plate is only loosely attached, an alternative proximal-to-distal method is preferred by some surgeons (Cordero's technique). A smooth curette (Freer septum elevator) is slid under the proximal nail fold and used to loosen the nail attachment by side-to-side movement; the removal is then continued in a distal direction.

Nail avulsion is an expedient treatment often used as a temporary measure to alleviate pain and discomfort in conditions such as ingrowing nail and acquired nail pachyonychia. It may also be done as part of a variety of biopsy techniques, involving partial or total nail removal which may be required for the exploration or removal of various nail tumours and infections.

Nail avulsion is a simple procedure, often dramatically relieving painful conditions, but it should not be used as a routine treatment since prolonged exposure of the nail bed may lead to permanent onycholysis, nail thickening or overcurvature.

Acute paronychia

Once pus formation has occurred in acute bacterial paronychia, surgical intervention is crucial to avoid permanent matrix damage and scarring. This is particularly so in young children.

If acute inflammatory signs do not remit within 2 days on appropriate oral antibiotic therapy, surgery is indicated since pus progressively tracks round the base of the nail. Incision should be carried out at the point of maximum tenderness or where pus is visibly localised. If this reveals a sinus track, its whole course should be exposed. Removal of the proximal third of the nail plate is recommended by many authorities to aid drainage and healing.

Chronic paronychia

Most cases of chronic paronychia (see p. 51) are slowly cured by avoidance of wetting, and treatment of the mixed microbial colonisation, for example with Daktacort (miconazole hydrocortisone) cream or equivalent. In a minority of cases conservative methods are not curative, and the infection and nail fold thickening progress. Two surgical techniques may help at this stage:

(1) Liquid nitrogen spray for approximately 20 seconds to the affected proximal and lateral nail folds.
(2) Excision of a crescent-shaped piece of full-thickness skin including the whole of the inflamed proximal nail fold (Fig. 13.3); after this procedure, regrowth of the nail folds and cuticle takes place in approximately 2 months.

Cryosurgery may cause temporary leukonychia (Fig. 13.4) or onychomadesis but heals within 2–3 weeks; proximal nail fold excision heals slowly but does not produce a nail dystrophy.

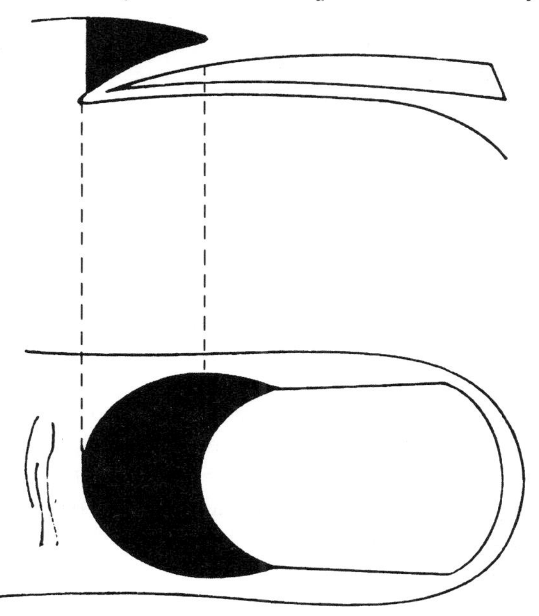

Fig. 13.3 Chronic paronychia: diagram showing (black) area to be removed in recalcitrant cases

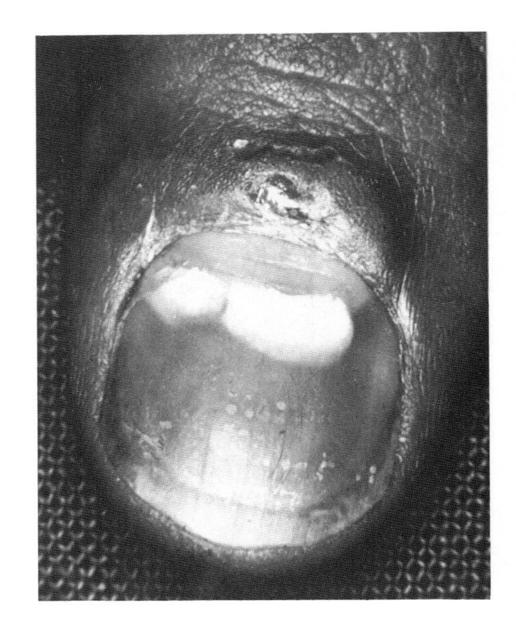

Fig. 13.4 Leukonychia after cryosurgery to the proximal nail fold

Cryosurgery

Traditionally, cryosurgery in the nail region has been reserved for treating periungual warts. Pain during and after treatment is the main disadvantage. This can be minimised by (1) pre-treatment local anaesthesia, or (2) oral aspirin 600 mg three times daily, commencing 2 hours before, and for 3 days after treatment, together with Dermovate (clobetasol propionate) cream applied twice daily until the acute inflammatory signs have subsided. Periungual warts are notoriously difficult to treat and cryosurgery is unlikely to effect cure without several repeat treatments, fortnightly. It should therefore be reserved for the most recalcitrant cases.

Successful treatment of myxoid cysts with liquid nitrogen spray cryosurgery has recently been described (Dawber *et al.*, 1983). The most promising technique involves pricking the cyst and expressing the gelatinous contents before spraying the cystic area, and 1 cm proximal to it, with liquid nitrogen spray. Permanent cure is obtained in over 80% of treated cases.

Cryosurgery has found a place in the treatment of many benign vascular lesions of the skin and mucous membranes, but there is as yet no evidence that similar success will be obtained for the treatment of equivalent lesions of the nail apparatus.

Carbon dioxide laser

The CO_2 laser destroys tissue by vaporisation within the treated area. The laser beam is narrow (0.1–0.2 mm) and since heat is not conducted away from the site of impact, there is little thermal damage to adjacent tissue. In nail pathology, the advantages of the CO_2 laser include good haemostasis, an antiseptic effect, accuracy of tissue killing, little thermal damage or postoperative pain, good healing and excellent cosmetic results. Good results have been obtained in the treatment of ingrowing toe nail, onychogryphosis and pyogenic granuloma.

Congenital and traumatic deformities

Malalignment of the matrix

In this dystrophy the nail matrix of the great toe is deviated laterally with respect to the longitudinal axis of the digit. This predisposes to painful traumatic damage particularly sited at the tip of the affected toe and ingrowing toe nail. A late consequence of malalignment is hemionychogryphosis. Corrective treatment involves rotating the whole nail apparatus medially to correct the matrix alignment (Fig. 13.5). This should ideally be done within the first 2 years of life in cases in which the deviation is marked.

Pachyonychia congenita

Should the affected nail be extremely hypertrophic in pachyonychia congenita, to preserve normal toe and finger function it may be necessary to remove the whole nail apparatus with grafting; or curettage and electrocautery or chemical cautery.

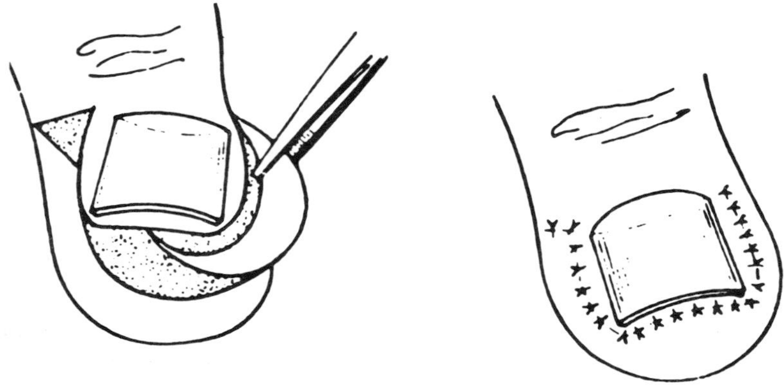

Fig. 13.5 Procedure to correct congenital malalignment of the big toe nail

Racket thumbs

A good cosmetic result can be obtained by bilateral nail narrowing. This involves removing a section of the nail apparatus adjacent to the lateral nail folds, similar to the longitudinal nail biopsy method of Zaias (1967).

The 'nail narrowing' operation may also be a suitable technique for the removal of longitudinal pigmented bands, ingrowing toe nail and longitudinal traumatic fissures.

Longitudinal fissures (split nail deformity)

Traumatic longitudinal fissures due to punctate matrix scarring, usually affecting only one nail, are relatively common and interfere with the normal function of the distal nail border and fingertip. This permanent split must be differentiated from Heller's median canaliform dystrophy (p. 99) which usually returns to normal after several years.

Surgical treatment of this scar is by exposure and excision, after reflecting back the proximal nail fold and avulsing the nail plate. Following elliptical excision of the scar the defect is sutured with 6/0 plain catgut. The trimmed nail should then be reapposed to the nail bed and sutured into position as a temporary covering. Laterally placed fissures are best removed by the technique similar to the lateral longitudinal biopsy—as for nail narrowing.

Narrow bands of post-traumatic pterygium may be corrected by the same method.

Ingrowing toe nail

Pain, infection, excessive granulation and overgrowth of the inflamed lateral nail folds are the main disabilities with ingrowing nail. While the early inflammatory phase may be arrested with antiseptic soaks and oral broad spectrum antibiotic treatment, many cases progress and require surgical intervention. Various techniques are available depending on the type of deformity and severity. Three major types can be defined: (1) subcutaneous ingrown nail—perforation of the nail groove epithelium by a spicule of nail plate; (2) hypertrophy of the lateral nail fold; (3) over-curvature of the nail plate—'pincer nail' deformity.

Early stage treatment should involve antiseptic soaks and careful exploration under local anaesthesia to define and remove any lateral nail spicules; a piece of cotton wool is then forced under the nail plate to prevent further lateral ingrowing as the nail plate moves distally.

Excessive inflammatory granulation tissue is a common complication of ingrowing toe nail. If this is accompanied by bacterial infection, liquid nitrogen spray cryosurgery may be successful—a single 20 second spray to induce ice formation in the granulation tissue and associated lateral nail fold. Soluble aspirin 600 mg three times daily for 3 days and clobetasol propionate cream twice daily to the treated area will minimise the immediate inflammatory reaction. In the absence of bacterial infection, removal of the granulation tissue by curettage and excision of the whole length of the lateral part of the nail plate (approximately one-fifth) is recommended. The area from which the granulation tissue has been removed may be treated by a silver nitrate pencil or liquid phenol. If relapse occurs, a permanent procedure may be required. A commonly used limited technique involves removal of the lateral matrix, corresponding to the lateral nail plate section previously removed.

If these conservative techniques fail or the presenting nail dystrophy is bilateral and incapacitating, total matrix removal

(Zadik procedure) or chemical ablation may be indicated. This is carried out after proximal nail fold reflection and nail removal. The Zadik operation should be reserved for severe cases or for failure with the more limited methods in view of the functional importance of the great toe nails.

For exact details of these surgical techniques the reader is referred to more detailed texts.

The pincer nail (over-curvature) deformity (Fig. 13.6) may be entirely asymptomatic, or painful due to inclusion of dermis and bone in the rolled nail, particularly if the great toe nail is affected. If pain is severe then surgery is indicated. If the patient is old, infirm or inactive, removal of the nail and matrix ablation is indicated.

Pain may be cured by the simple expedient of clipping the infolded lateral edges as proximally as possible, under local anaesthetic if necessary. Some centres have devised nail braces (orthonyx) to fit the over-curved nails exactly and impart pull to flatten the nail plate—this process may take up to 6 months to be effective.

If the pain is specifically associated with the lateral curvature, bilateral lateral nail resection, as for ingrowing toe nail, should be carried out together with lateral matrix resection.

More detailed techniques are available when the rolled nail encloses bone and soft tissues; these will not be considered here.

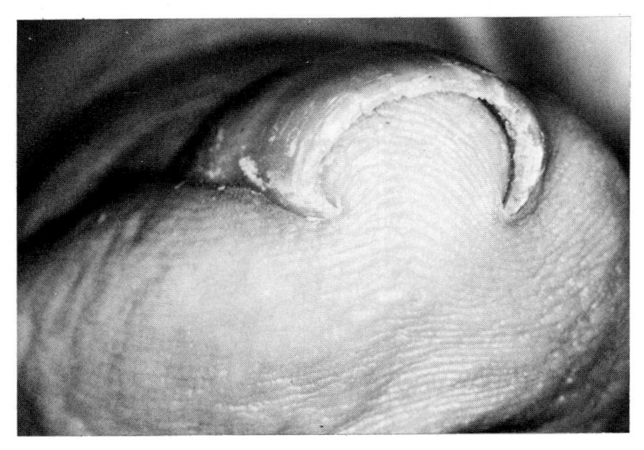

Fig. 13.6 Pincer nail deformity

Onychogryphosis

Onychogryphosis is an acquired hypertrophy particularly affecting the great toe nails, which is most commonly seen in the old or infirm patient; a previous history of nail trauma may be obtained and hallux valgus is often an associated sign. Once the nail becomes grossly thickened and deformed, cutting becomes a problem since household nail scissors and clippers are inadequate. The nail may grow in a coiled fashion and resemble a ram's horn.

If there is peripheral vascular disease or diabetes then conservative techniques using electric drills and burrs may be employed to thin the thickened nail plate. Regular clipping will then be necessary to prevent relapse. In the presence of good vascular supply, removal of the hypertrophied nail plate is indicated, followed by total matrix ablation. Anecdotal reports have recently appeared suggesting that CO_2 laser treatment gives good results.

References

Bureau, H, Baran, R and Haneke, E (1984) Nail surgery and traumatic abnormalities. In *Diseases of the Nail and their Management*, eds Baran, R and Dawber, R P R. Chapter 11, pp. 347–402, Oxford: Blackwell.

Dawber, R P R, Sonnex, T, Leonard, J and Ralfs, I (1983) Myxoid cyst of the finger: treatment by liquid nitrogen spray cryosurgery. *Clin. Exp. Derm.* **8** 153

Scher, R and Ackerman, A B (1980) Subtle clues to diagnosis from biopsies of nails. Histological differential diagnosis of onychomycosis and psoriasis of the nail unit from cornified cells of the nail bed alone. *Amer. J. Dermatopathol.* **2(3)** 255

Zaias, N (1967) The longitudinal nail biopsy. *J. Invest. Derm.* **49** 406

Appendix

Glossary of terms used in nail diseases

Acaulosis unguis	Infection of nail with *Scopulariopsis brevicaulis*
Agnail	Hang nail; hard spicules at edge of nail
Anonychia	Absence of the nail
Defluvium unguium	Nail shedding, starting at base and extending forward
Fragilitas unguium	Brittle nails
Hapalonychia	Soft nails
Koilonychia	Spoon-shaped nails
Leukonychia	White nails
Lunula	Pale area at base of nail often called the half-moon and is the exposed part of the nail matrix
Macronychia	Large but otherwise normal nails
Micronychia	Small but otherwise normal nails
Onychalgia nervosa	Exquisitely sensitive nails
Onychauxis	Hypertrophied nails
Onychia	Inflammation of nail either post-traumatic or with paronychia
Onychodysplasia	Abnormal development or growth of nail
Onychogryphosis	Long, thick and curved nail
Onychoheterotrophia	Misplaced nails
Onycholysis	Separation of nail from its bed
Onychomadesis	Nail shedding starting at base and extending forward (same as defluvium unguium)
Onychomycosis	Fungal infection of nail plate
Onychophagia	Nail biting
Onychorrhexis	Excess longitudinal striation
Onychoschizia	Splitting of nails into layers

Onychotillomania	Picking at a nail from habit
Pachyonychia	Thickening of nail usually increasing from base to tip
Panaritium	Abscess at side or base of nail (whitlow)
Paronychia	Inflammation of tissues surrounding the nail
Platonychia	Increased curvature in long axis
Polyonychia	Two or more separate nails on one digit
Pterygium unguis	Overgrowth of cuticle on to nail eventually destroying nail
Trachyonychia	Rough nails
Unguis incarnatus	Ingrowing nail
Usure des ongles	Wearing away of nails due to scratching

Index